Comprehensive Outline of Microbiological Diseases

Perry Haalman

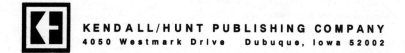

KENDALL/HUNT PUBLISHING COMPANY
4050 Westmark Drive   Dubuque, Iowa 52002

Dedicated

To My Wife

Michele M. Haalman

Whose patience is unimaginable
Whose kindness knows no bounds
A spouse that very few husbands have the opportunity to know
Let alone marry

To her my many thanks

CONTENTS

i

This book is an outline, a skeleton of information, regarding microbiological diseases. It is meant to help you organize the immense amount of information about diseases into some form useful to your chosen profession.

NOTE: It is important to say the name of diseases and causative agents out loud so you become familiar with the words and their usage.

It is important that this book does not replace classroom or practical experience. This is the reason for the space provided for notes. By taking notes in class and adding material as you work you create a very useful and personal reference work. In a word you will put the flesh on the bones.

Early in this experience, memorization will be important, but you must recognize that eventually the material must become second nature to you if you are to succeed in clinical medicine, for microbiological diseases are still a major killer of the patients we treat.

I would like to thank Carol and Georgeann for their untiring efforts in deciphering my non-legible writing and producing the manuscript for this text. A herculean task done with grace, elegance and perseverance. I also would like to thank Lori Crowel for her excellent illustrations, which are almost photographic in their execution. Chris Schenk, Associate Editor, Kendall Hunt, deserves my thanks for his patience and help in the management of the "nitty-gritty" aspects of publishing this book.

However, in the final analysis, it is my work. Any errors, by omission or commission are my own. I stand corrected where they may occur and would appreciate knowing about them. I hope the purchaser of this book finds it useful.

December, 1993

Perry Haalman

VIRAL DISEASES
ACQUIRED VIA THE RESPIRATORY ROUTE

short incubation {

Common cold
Parainfluenza Viral Disease
Croup
Adenoviral Disease
Influenza

Long incubation {

Mumps
Measles
Rubella
Chickenpox
Shingles
Smallpox
Roseola infantum
Molluscum contagiosum
Fifth Disease

NAME OF DISEASE: Common cold
OTHER NAME(S):   Acute coryza, Afebrile respiratory disease

Causative Agent: Rhinovirus

Characteristics of Organism:
     Picornavirus
     Over 100 antigenic types
     Viral particle - 15-30 nanometers
     Cytopathic effect - plaques of dead cells
     Resistant to disinfectants
     Sensitive to acids
     Other virus involved include
          Coronavirus effects epithelium, acute respiratory distress, pneumonia-like
          Myxovirus, adenovirus, coxsackievirus, echovirus

Portal of Entry:
     Respiratory Route -   Nasopharyrgael secretions droplet spray
     Indirect (fomites) -   contaminated hands

Clinical Symptoms:
     Incubation two to four days
     Pharyngitis/increased watery discharge
     Coryza
     Headache
     nonproductive cough/sneezing
     Lacrimation
     Fever/chills
     Duration three to six days (Infectious first two to three days)

Complications:
     Bacterial otitis media   *middle ear infection*
     Bacterial pneumonia - very young or very old

Diagnosis:
>   Rare
>   Organism can be grown on tissue culture
>   Monolayer of human embryo or primary
>   Monkey kidney tissue
>   Needs high oxygen concentration
>>   neutral ph
>>   temperature ~33°C

Treatment:
>   Aspirin/Acetaminophen - fever/pains
>   Liquids - dehydration
>   Rest

Epidemiology:
>   Vaccine impractical - various antigenic strains
>   Immunity via IgA - general - two months
>>   specific two years

No cures

NAME OF DISEASE: Parainfluenza Respiratory Disease
OTHER NAME(S):   Parainfluenza

Causative Organism: Parainfluenza virus

Characteristics of Organism:
    Paramyxovirus ~100 to 300 nanometers
    Enveloped/sensitive
    Non-segmented genome
    Spherical
    ssRNA *-spikes*
    Hemagglutinin/Neuraminidase
    Cytopathic effect - giant cell formation
    Serotypes - 1,2,3,4A,4B
        Type 1a (sub of 4) = Sendai
        Type 3 = 1 (hemabsorption)
        Type 2 = CA (Croup-associated)
        Type 1 = HA 2
    Sensitive drying
        Disinfectants
        Temperature extremes

Portal of Entry:
    Respiratory Route

Symptoms:
    Incubation period three to six days
    fever/chills
    cough/nasal discharge
    reddened throat
    Upper respiratory in children
    Low respiratory in adults

Diagnosis:
    Serology - Hemadsorpton of guinea pig RBC's
    Grows on Rhesus monkey kidney tissue culture and amniotic sac of chick embryo tissue culture (seven to nine days old)

Treatment:
    Symptomatic

Epidemiology:
    Formalin inactivated polyvalent vaccine
    Against 1,2,3

NAME OF DISEASE: Croup
OTHER NAME(S):   Acute laryngotracheobronchitis

Causative Organism: Respiratory syncytial virus also called
pneumovirus

Characteristics of Organism:
    Paramyxovirus
    Two serotypes - A and B
    Enveloped/sensitive
    Cytopathic effect - syncytium formation
                Intracytoplasmic inclusions
                No Hemagglutinin/Neuraminidase

Portal of Entry:
    Respiratory route

Clinical symptoms:
    Incubation four to five days
    Three groups base on severity

    First group -   cough/hoarseness
                    rhinitis/pharyngitis
                    otitis
                    stridor (high pitched breathing)

    Second group -   Fever
                    Toxemia
                    Dyspnea/wheezing
                    rales

    Third group -   Convulsions
                    Cyanosis
                    Dehydration
                    Restlessness

Complications: Otitis media
                    Necotrizing bronchitis
                    Bronchiolitis
                    Interstitial pneumonia
                    Tracheal obstruction

Handwritten notes in margin: cry Aloud; RS:; BARking's cough; respiratory failure; RT side heart failure

Diagnosis:

    Specimens -   sputum

                           Tracheal washing

    Culture -   chicken embryo tissue culture

    Serology -   ELISA

                           Indirect immunofluorescent test

Epidemiology:

    Most severe under six months old. Mother's antibodies are

          no protection

    Late winter/early spring

    Males affected more that females

NAME OF DISEASE: Adenoviral Diseases
OTHER NAME(S):   APC diseases
                  (adenoidal, pharyngeal, conjunctival diseases)

Causative Organism: Adenovirus

Characteristics of Organism:
    Adenovirus
    cubical/nonenveloped
    Capsid 60 - 90 nanometers
    252 capsomeres/capsid
    ds DNA
    Stable and survives long time in environment
    47 antigenic types identified by numbers
    Slow, erratic growth patterns
    Cytopathic effects - hosts cells swell to form grape-like
        clusters
    Intranuclear inclusions
                Cowdry type
                Smudge type

Portal of Entry:
    Respiratory Route
    Direct contact (conjunctiva)

Clinical Symptoms:
    1.   Acute Febrile respiratory illness (AFRI)
            Children -   cough/sore throat
                          Nasal secretions
                          headache
                          fever
    2.   Acute respiratory disease (ARD)
            Adults -   Resembles flu
                          Virus 3, 4, 7, 7a
                          Fever
                          dry cough/sore throat
                          minimal sputum
                          anorexia
                          Vaccine used in military

8

3. Acute pharyngoconjunctival fever (APF)
                      Spiking fever
                      sore throat
                      Follicular conjunctivitis
                      Viruses 3, 4, 7, 14

4. Acute Epidemic Kertoconjunctivities (AEK)
                      incubation 5 - 7 days
                      follicular conjunctivitis
                      conjunctival edema
                      blurred vision/photophobia
                      virus 8
                      pools, instruments etc.
                      could lead to impaired vision

5. Hemorrhagic cystitis
        Boys -   hematuria   — Blood
                      urinary frequency
                      dysuria

Complications:
      Meningitis (virus 7)
      Gastroententis
      Necrotizing bronchitis
      bronchiolitis - necrosis/desquamation
                      epithelium
                          debris - epithelial cells, mucus,
                                   mono-nuclear cells
                      bronchiole like-
                      thrombosed vessels

                  Interstitial pneumonia - consolidation
                                           necrosis
                                           hemorrhage
                                           edema

Diagnosis:
   Isolated from sputum, conjunctival secretions, stool

   Culture - Hela cell culture, human embryo tissue culture

   Serology   - complement - fixation
                neutralization tests

Treatment:
   Symptomatic

Epidemiology:
   Some adenovisuses considered oncogenic
   strongly types 12, 18, 31
   mildly types 3, 7, 14, 16, 21

NAME OF DISEASE: Influenza
OTHER NAME(S):   Flu, grippe

Causative Organism: Influenza virus

Characteristics of Organism:
    Orthromyxovirus
    Helical enveloped - ether sensitive
    80-180 nanometers
    ssRNA / segmented - 8 pieces   *LARGE SPIKES*
    Prominent spikes - 10-14 nanometers
    2 protein components of capsid (peplomers)
    3 types hemagglutinin, main function not to agglutinate   *← Important to classification*
        RBC's but to attach to host mucosa
    2 types neuraminidase - dissolves
        mucous on mucosa
        assist in budding
        host cell fusion
    2 antigens -   S = nucleocapsid
                      M = protein of envelop
    Cytopathic effect - destruction of cilia

Portal of Entry:
    Respiratory

Clinical Symptoms:
    Uncomplicated
        Incubation 1 to 3 days
        ✓ Anorexia - *lost of Appetite*
        ✓ Insomnia - *can't sleep*
        ✓ Muscles pain (back/legs)
        ✓ Photophobia
        Fever - 101 - 104°F
        Dry cough/sore throat
    Complicated (Fatal)
        Predisposition -   Age
                            Cardio-respiratory disease
                            Severe inflammatory edema
        Bronchiolus thicken, distend
        Mononuclear infiltration

11

NOTES:

Ciliated epithelium and goblet cells destroyed
Diffuse necrotizing hemorrhagic pneumonitis
Necrotizing Bronchitis
Macrophage inhibition - impaired immunity
Cyanosis/dypnea
Little or no pleurisy
Respiratory Failure

Complications:

Secondary bacterial infection
particularly respiratory involving

Staphylococcus aureus
Streptococcus pneumonia

Evidence - pleurisy
bloody sputum

Diagnosis:

Clinical - patient's symptoms
Cultural - isolate virus
grows in allantoic and ammoniac space of fertile hen's egg
Serology - Immunofluorescent Test
Hemaglutimation inhibition Test
Complement Fixation

Treatment:

Uncomplicated - Symptomatic
Complicated -
Type A - Amantadine HCl (Symmetrel)
Interfere with uncoating of virus
Type A and B - Ribavirin

Epidemiology:

3 Antigenic strains
Type A - first isolated 1933
named "A Classic"
changes antigenicity regularly
due to antigenic drift = mutations
antigenic shift = recombination
(two types in one host)

exchange of genetic

1947 - Type A_1 (prime)
1957 - Type A_2 (asian)
1968 - Type A_3 (hong kong)
Nomenclature
(example) A/H. K./1-68/H_3/N_2
or A/USSR/90-77/H_1/N_1
Implicated in epidemic/pandemic of 1917-
1918 - Type A (swine)

Type B First isolated in 1940
Antigenically more stable
Only has antigen drift for variability

Type C First isolated in 1947
Antigenically stable
No Neuraminidase - reason not
involved in disease

Influenza among top 10 killers of citizens in the United States.

Vaccine available - changed yearly for anticipated
strains, formalin/inactivated, chicken embryo
Side effects - virus/vaccine
Guillaine - Barre Syndrome
Ascending paralysis
Muscular pain/weakness
Reyes's Syndrome
Prolonged vomiting
high fever
convulsion
liver damage - fatty infiltration
edema of brain
Associated more with Type B
Newest vaccine - split vaccine
Hemaglutinin spikes given separately from
neuraminidase spikes
One month later neuraminidase spikes

NAME OF DISEASE: Mumps
OTHER NAME(S):   Infectious parotitis, contagious parotitis, epidemic parotitis, parotitis epidemica

Causative Organism: Mumps virus

Characteristics of Organism:
    Paramyxovirus
        helical/enveloped - ether sensitive
        ssRNA
    Agglutinates blood
        Two antigens S and D
        Hemolytic activity - weak

Portal of Entry:
    Respiratory route
        via saliva - direct
        indirect-fomites
        urine also infectious

Clinical symptoms:
    Incubation - 14 to 25 days (average 16-18)
        Infectious for 7 days before appearance of symptoms
        Swelling of parotid glands
        bilateral/unilateral
        Dysphagia
        Fever 101°-104°F
        earache
        Parotid exhibits interstitial edema and inflammation - infiltration with hisocytes, lymphocytes, plasma cells
        compression of acini ducts

Complications:
    orchitis/epididymitis - usually unilateral
    painful swelling of tissue
        atrophy
        sterility rare

oophoritis - enlarged ovaries
back pain
sterility rare
acute pancreatitis - beta cells and pancreatic cells affected
meningitis, fever, headache, vomiting,
nausea, stiff neck
deafness usually unilateral
encephalitis

Diagnosis:
    Clinical picture
    Culture -   virus from saliva - urine
                  on chicken embryo (amniotic cavity)
                  monkey kidney or human heteroploidic
                  epithelial tissue culture
    serology -   four-fold increase antibody titre in blood
                  skin sensitivity test

Treatment:
    Symptomatic
    Gamma globulin in pre-pubescent boys prevents orchitis

Epidemiology:
    Vaccine   Live, attenuated strain
                  Grown in duck embryo
                  (Jenny Lynn)
                  Administered with measles
                  and rubella (MMR vaccine)
                  Introduced - 1967
                  Within first 10 years a 10 fold reduction in
                  the number of mumps cases - indication of
                  effectiveness

NAME OF DISEASE: **Measles**
OTHER NAME(S):   **Rubeola, morbilli, red measles, 14-day measles, hard measles**

Causative Organism: **Measles virus**

Characteristics of Organism:
        Paramyxovirus
        helical/enveloped, ether sensitive
        ssRNA
        non-segment genome
        Cytopathic effect -   giant cells
                                  inclusion bodies

Portal of Entry:
        Respiratory route
            via saliva
            urine also infectious

Clinical Symptoms:
        Incubation   10 - 14 days
                      (Infectious before symptoms appear)

        Two stages
            Prodromal stage
                high fever - 104°-105°F
                    hacking dry cough
                    sinusitis
                    tracheobronchitis
                    Koplik spots - diagnostically
                    significant - bluish -   white dots
                                        red halo
                                        1 - 3 millimeters
                    buccal mucosa near molars
      1st stage — Koplik spots result from
                    epithelial giant cells with
                    intranuclear inclusions

Exanthem (rash) stage
    Erythematous maculopapular rash
    Relation of T-cells and viral
    infected cells in same blood vessels
    first on forehead/behind ears
    spreads downward and out
    fades - leaving a brownish discoloration
Effected skin -   dilated epithelial
                vesicles
                edema
                mononuclear cell infiltrate
Lymphatic tissue - Follicular hyperplasia
                Worthin - Finkeldey
                Giant - Cells
                      100 + nuclei
                      intranuclear and
                      intracytoplasmic inclusions

Course of disease:
    Virus to lymphoid tissue of tonsils, adenoids
    via lymph
    RES - hyperplasia - leucopenia
    to blood and body

Complications:
    Otitis media
    bronchopneumonia
    Viral encephalitis
    Subacute Sclerosing Panencephalitis (SSPE)
        1 in 10,000
        Degeneration of nervous system
            first intellectual skills
            then cortical
            Death
    Part of CHINA - Chronic infectious neuropathic agents
        mortality - about 30%
        permanent damage - 1/3

brain disease 1-2 years after disease

17

Diagnosis:
>   Clinical picture
>   Microscopic - basal cell mucosal smear
>   Serology -   hemagglutination - inhibition
>   complement fixation

Treatment:
>   Symptomatic
>   children under 3 - prophylactic antibiotics

Epidemiology:
>   Part of MMR vaccine
>   Introduced 1964
>   various problems - various forms of vaccine
>   1st Edmonston - live attenuated vaccine
>   Grown -   monkey kidney
>   human amnion
>   chicken embryo
>   High incidence of fever and exanthematous reaction
>   Modified with gamma - globulin
>   3rd type FAV (further attenuated
>   vaccine, United Kingdom vaccine)
>
>   Also killed (formaldehyde) vaccine
>   If measle afterward develop
>   Atypical measles -   pneumonitis
>   pinpoint blisters/rash
>   hemorrhages
>   self - recovering
>   hypersensitivity reaction

Treat symptoms

Severe forms uses

18

NAME OF DISEASE: Rubella
OTHER NAME(S):   German measles, three-day measles, soft measles

Causative Organism: Rubella virus

Characteristics of Organism:
    Togavirus
    40-80 nanometers
    ss RNA
    Cubic/non - enveloped
    hemagglutinin - negative
    cytopathic effect - difficult to detect

Portal of Entry:
    Respiratory route -
        nasal secretions highly infectious

Clinical Symptoms
    Incubation - 14 - 21 days (average 16-18)
        infectious before symptoms

    Two stages
    Prodromal stage
        low grade fever
        headache
        conjunctivitis
        rhinitis
        suborbipital, post auricular,
        postcervical lymphadenopathy

    Exanthem rash stage
        Begins on face
        maculopapular rash
        red, petechial, macular rash or soft palate - Forschheimer spots

    Young females, post pubescent transient arthritis

Complications:
    During 1ˢᵗ trimester crosses placenta
    slows cellular movements - effects fetus
    (Synchronization, specialization, differentiation effected)

cataract	bone abnormalities
deafness	microcephaly
retardation	pigmentary retinopathy
anemia	septal heart defects
thrombocytopenia	abortion
tetralogy of fallot	

Diagnosis:
    Clinical picture
    Serology - four fold increase in antibody titre
    Culture virus

Treatment:
    Symptomatic

Epidemiology:
    Vaccine   Introduced in 1969
        Contro - indicated pregnant women
         side effects - fever, rash transient arthritis
    Rubella part of TORHCH group of diseases which affect
        fetuses and newborns

NOTES:

NAME OF DISEASE: Chicken pox
OTHER NAME(S):   Varicella   — *Tiny spot*

Causative Organism: herpes varicella - zoster virus or V-Z
                     virus

Characteristic of Organism:
        Herpetovirus
        ds DNA
        Cubic 162 capsomere
        Cytopathic effect   multinucleated giant cells
                            ballooning of epithelial cells
                            Type A cowdry inclusion   *Spike*
                            body - acidophilic
                            (eosinophilic) intranuclear
                            inclusion, ½ size of
                            nucleus, clear zone or halo

Portal of Entry:
        Respiratory -   direct
                               indirect
        Incubation -   14 to 17 days
                  not contagious 7 or more days after eruption
        Two stages
        Prodromal   low fever
                               vague pains   *Not like flu*
                               beginnings of macular rash   *Just don't feel well*
                               lasts about 24 hours   *abdomen - rash*
        Vesicle stage   Macular rash changes to papular   *crops*
                               Papular to clear vesicles on
                               erythematous base
                               vesicles cloud, break, scab
                               new crops every 3 or 4 days
                               Damage to cells of small blood
                               vessels and lymphatics -
                               thromboses/hemorrhage

21

Course of Disease:
>   Nasopharynx to viremia
>   To RES
> 2nd wave viremia from RES
>   Lead to rash and vesicles

Complications:
>   Encephalitis
>   Hepatitis
>   Myositis
>   Keratitis
>   Myocarditis
>   Pneumonia - death due to damaged vessels
>   With children salicyletis can result in
>>   Reyes Syndrome
>>   acute encelopathy
>>   fatty infiltration/degeneration of liver, spleen, kidney

associated w/ Reyes syndrom

Diagnosis:
>   Clinical picture
>   Microscopic (to distinguish small pox, no need today)
>>   Cellular smear
>>   Giemsa stain
>>   observe inclusions
>   Serology   Complement Fixation
>>   Fluorescent antibody test

Treatment:
>   Symptomatic
>   Early, particularly comprised patient pooled gamma globulin
>
>   Steroids contra-indicated - increase severity
>   For encephalitis-adenine arabinoside
>   (ARA-A)

No steroids

Epidemiology:
>   Vaccine   live, attenuated vaccine
>>   approved
>>   Given with MMR
>   Over 2,000,000 cases per year, second to gonorrhea in list
>   of infectious diseases

usually you have chicken pox first

NAME OF DISEASE: Shingles
OTHER NAME(S):   Zoster

Causative Organism: V-Z virus

Characteristics of Organism:
    See chickenpox

Portal of Entry:
    Latent infection
    virus hides in cervical or sacral root ganglia

More woman Facially - men red welt pox females - abdomen

Clinical Picture:
    Fever/malaise
    pain over body (hyper or paresthesia)
    In about 2 weeks - red nodular lesion
    erupt thin - walled, fluid - filled vesicles
    Rupture/scab
    Suitable environment secondary
    bacterial infections
    Nerve damage necrosis
    Convalescence - extensive time
    Persistent Pain - post - zoster neuralgia

Course of Disease:
    Lack of suitable antibodies or
    predisposition (stress, malnutrition)
    virus multiply in ganglia
    cause necrosis
    Spread down sensory nerves
    Frequently facial nerves
        5-7TH intercostal nerves

As you get older

Women more than men under BRA.

Complications:
    Primarily secondary bacterial infections

Diagnosis:
    Clinical picture
    Spinal tap increased pressure
                increased protein

Treatment:
    Asymptomatic
    Alleviate pain
    Sterile maintenance of infected region

NAME OF DISEASE: Smallpox
OTHER NAME(S):   Variola

Causative Organism: Poxvirus variola

Characteristics of Organism:
      Poxvirus
      Elliptical or globular shape
      280 x 220 globular shape
      non-enveloped
      swirling fibers on nucleocapsid
      cytopathic effect - syncytial formation
                          cell clumping
                          guaneri body
                          inclusions - acidophilic
                          cytoplasmic
      Grown on tissue culture -
                          human epithelium
                          HelLa cells
                          CAM of Fertilized
                          hen's egg

Portal of Entry:
      Respiratory route
      Body secretions

Clinical Symptoms:
      Incubation   high fever - 104°F
                          severe chills
                          headache/backache
                          prostration
                          stupor/coma
      Rash stage   macular rash usually forehead
                          changes to papular
                          to vesicular to pustular
                          pustules very large
                          rupture, scab
                          emit pus, soft scar
                          becomes a pock

Complication:

Secondary   bacterial infections
                abscesses
                carbuncles
                osteomyelitis

Diagnosis:

Serology -   Increasing titre
Four tests -   electron microscopy
                growth on CAM-grey-white pocks
                agar-gel precipitation
                tissue culture

Treatment:

N-methy-lisatin beta-thio-semcarbazone

Epidemiology:

Vaccine   oldest, introduced by Jenner
              no longer used
              smallpox eradicated as of October 26, 1979

NAME OF DISEASE: Roseola infantum
OTHER NAME(S):   Exanthem subitem, roseola subitem
pseudorubella, rose-spots

Causative Organism: Not isolated

Portal of Entry:
    Not determined

Clinical Symptoms:
    Incubation - 7 to 17 days
    High fever - 104-105°F, sudden on-set
    Convulsions/seizures
    In 3-5 days fever drops
    Rash after fever
    Fine, macular rash, blanches on pressure
    Erythematous streaks on palate

Diagnosis:
    Clinical picture - rash disappears in 48 hours

Epidemiology:
    Mostly 6 months - 3 year old children

NAME OF DISEASE: Molluscum contagiosum

Causative Organism: Molluscum contagiosum virus

Characteristics of Organism:
    Pox virus
    Large, elliptical shape
    Cytopathic effect - acidophilic, cytoplasmic
                inclusions - Mollosucum bodies

Portal of Entry:
    Direct contact (children)
    sexual (adults)

Clinical Picture:
    Incubation - 2 to 8 weeks
    Small papillomatous lesion at site of inoculation - pink,
        wart-like (face, buttocks, extremities)
    Firm, waxy, elevated with depressed center
    Milky curd release when pressed
    Lesion itch, painful

Diagnosis:
    Microscopic - Skin slides -   balloning degeneration
                                      acanthosis
                                      hyperplasia
                                      Molluscum bodies

Treatment:
    Excision/Curettement

NAME OF DISEASE: Fifth Disease
OTHER NAME(S):   Erythema infectiosum

Causative Organism: Parvo virus B 19

Characteristics of Organism:
    ss DNA
    cubic -   23-32 capsomere
               defective
    non-enveloped

Portal of Entry:
    Respiratory Route

Clinical Symptoms:
    low grade fever
    rash on cheeks/abdomen
    destroys RBC's stem cells

    Congenital - fatal anemia

Small virus

Incubation could be weeks

heat /

VIRAL DISEASE

VIA

GASTROINTESTINAL ROUTE

Poliomyelitis
Coxsackie Viral Diseases
Echo Viral Diseases
Infectious Hepatitis
Hepatitis E
Infectious Mononucleosis

gray matter

NAME OF DISEASE: Poliomyelitis
OTHER NAME(S):   Polio, Infantile Paralysis

Causative Organism: Poliovirus

Characteristics of Organism:
    Picornavirus
        subdivision - enteroviruses
    ssRNA
    Cubical, non-enveloped
    27 nanometers with 32 capsomeres
    Three antigenic types cause disease
        Type 1 -   Brunhilde (Mahoney)
        Type 2 -   Lansing
        Type 3 -   Leon   *- serious problem in vaccine*
    Other antigen types do not cause disease
    Tissue cultured in Hela cells or diploid monkey kidney cells

Portal of Entry: Fecal-oral route -   contaminated water
                                pharyngeal secretions

Cl_2 kill polio virus

Predispositions: Age
                Pregnancy
                Excessive muscular activity
                Localized trauma

Clinical Symptoms:
    1. Asymptomatic - carrier
                    human body host
    2. Abortive (non-paralytic) poliomyelitis
                    Incubation - 5-35 days (7-14 average)
                    Low-grade fever
                    Malaise
                    Headache
                    Sore throat
                    Drowsiness
                    Nausea/vomiting
                    Resembles flu - "Summer Flu"

contagious

like Flu

31

3. Paralytic poliomyelitis - two varieties
     Motor (spinal) poliomyelitis
               Moderate fever
               headache
               Lethargy
               Vomiting
               Irritability
               Pain in neck, back, extremities
          Followed by a flaccid ascending
               paralysis - degree determined by
               where infection localized, cervical,
               thoracic, lumbar, affects motor
               neurons
               Abdominal distention
               Urinary retention
               Constipation
     Bulbar poliomyelitis - most severe
               Brain - stem infected
               Affects cranial nerves, particular 9-10
               Autonomic functions affected
               Symptoms of encephalitis
               Difficulty swallowing
               Regurgitation
               Respiratory distress -
                   pulmonary edema
                   shock

Course of disease:
    Ingestion
    Primary infection throat/small intestines
    Virus multiplies
    Invades lymphatic tissue - tonsils and peyer's patches
    Enters blood - viremia
        transient - progress no further
        persistent - penetrate capillary walls - Enter CNS

Diagnosis:

     Clinical picture

     Isolate virus - throat washings/stool

     Spinal tap - lymphocytosis

     Serology - four-fold increase in antibody titre - convalescent versus acute serum

Treatment:

     Minor forms - bed rest

     Major forms - non-paralytic - symptomatic

                paralytic - physical therapy
                          orthopedic apparati

                bulbar - use of Drinker's respirator (iron lung)
                        physical therapy
                        mental therapy

Epidemiology:

     Two vaccines:

        Salk - introduced 1955 (IPV, injectable polio vaccine)
            Formaldehyde inactivated virus
            Grown on monkey kidney tissue
            Series of 3 intra-muscular injections
            First three monovalent (MIPV)
            Six weeks apart
            Six month-trivalent duster (TIPV)
            Does not prevent infection
            Reduces incidence of paralysis

       Sabin Vaccine (OPV, oral polio vaccine)
            Two forms TOPU (trivalent)
            MOPV (monovalent) - TOPV preferred
            Two oral doses - 4-6 weeks apart
            6 months - 3rd dose
            Contains - live attenuated virus cultured in human cells
            Administered with DPT

     Vaccines have reduced the incidence from 10,000-15,0000/year to 100 or less/year

33

[handwritten notes in margin: "should give IPV before OPV", "vaccine type 1 2 3", "Prevents paralysis", "live virus", "< 1 Doz."]

Issue -   Reversion of Type 3 to wild type in OPV - can
                cause disease
         Risk greater than getting polio naturally acquired
        Solution -
            E-IPV with DPT - first time
            Followed by OPV

34

NAME OF DISEASE: Coxsackie viral diseases

Causative Organism: Coxsackie virus

Characteristics of Organism:
    Picornavirus
        Subdivision - enterovirus
    ssRNA
    Cubical/non-enveloped
    27 nanometers/32 capsomeres
    Two major antigenic groups
        Group A -   24 serotypes
                     degeneration of skeletal muscle
        Group B -   6 serotypes
                     inflammatory lesions
                         brain
                         heart
                         liver
                         pancreas
                         fat pads

Portal of Entry: Fecal - Oral route
    Group A diseases
        Paralytic illness -   resembles poliomyelitis
                                   (abortive)
        Aseptic meningitis -   stiff neck
                                   headache
                                   low-grade fever
                                   spontaneously recovering
        Herpengia -   Resembles flu
                       Children - 10 or under
                       Incubation - 2 to 9 days
                       Fever - 100°-104°F
                       Anorexia
                       Vomiting
                       Prostration
                       Dysphagia - multiple grayish - white
                           papulo-vesicular lesions on soft
                           palate and elsewhere in
                           oropharynx (1-2 millimeters)

→ swimming in contaminated H₂O

won·t die

35

Diarrhea
Muscle pain
Lasts 2 to 3 days

Group B Diseases
Pleurodynia (Devils grip, Bornholm disease)
Low grade fever
Pleuritic pain
Headache
Malaise
Aseptic meningitis
Epidemic myocarditis - infant
Associate with juvenile - onset diabetes

Diagnosis: Fecal washing
Serology -   Neutralization tests
Hemagglutination tests

Treatment: Symptomatic

Epidemiology:
Patient isolation
Nasal secretions
Fecal matter
Urine
All are contagious

No animal reservoir

NOTES:

NAME OF DISEASE: Echo Viral Diseases

Causative Organism: Echo Virus
                        (Enteric cytopathic human orphan)

found in gut

Characteristics of Organism:
        Picornavirus
                Subdivision - enterovirus
                ssRNA virus
                25-30 nanometers
                Cubical - 32 capsomeres
                Non-enveloped
                36 serotypes
                Cultured - monkey kidney or human amnion tissue

Portal of Entry: Fecal Oral Route

Clinical Symptoms:
        Neonatal Epidemic diarrhea
                severe diarrhea
                vomiting
                prefrontal headaches
                usually in nurseries, in summer
                Protection - breast feeding
        Aseptic meningitis
                flaccid paralysis
                types 2, 4, 6, 9, 16 involved
        Exanthems - maculopapular rash
                        (face - neck)
                        Spreads to body
                        Non-pruritic
                        Recovery 1-3 days
        Summer grippe - resembles flu

— Usually in Nurseries

like coxsackie Boston Diseases like Flu

Diagnosis:
        Serology -   Hemagglutination
                     Neutralization
                     (Four-fold increase in titre)

Treatment: Symptomatic

37

Epidemiology:
- Other diarrheal virus - infants
    - Norwalk like agent
        - ssRNA virus (calicivirus)
        - Contaminate food/water
        - Diarrhea/vomiting - short duration
        - Dehydration rare
    - Norwalk agent
        - Parvovirus
        - 24-48 hr incubation
        - Severe diarrhea
    - Rotavirus
        - Cubical, double-walled virus
        - Wheel shape
        - 11 segments to ds RNA
        - Nosocomial infection
        - Peak infection - 7-24 months old
        - Watery diarrhea
            - dehydration
            - vomiting
            - high fever - last

All multiply in epithelium lining of villi of small intestines
Non-specific inflammation
- Cytoplasmic vacuolization
- patchy mononuclear infiltrate
- erosion of villi
- lysis of epithelial cells

More severe effects liver

NAME OF DISEASE: Infectious hepatitis
OTHER NAME(S):   Viral Hepatitis A, Epidemic Jaundice, Catarrhal Jaundice, Short-incubation hepatitis

Causative Organism: Hepatitis A Virus (HAV)

Characteristics of Organism:
Picornavirus
    subdivision - enterovirus
ss RNA
Cubical/non-enveloped
25-30 nanometers, 32 capsomeres
Resistant to physical/chemical agents

Portal of Entry: Fecal - Oral Route
contaminated water
contaminated shellfish

Clinical Symptoms:
Incubation - 14-40 days   *< 30 days*
Fever - about 104°F
Diarrhea/nausea
Headache
Cervical lymph node enlargement
Appendicitis-like pain   *- VAgus nerve*
Dark urine
Clay-colored stools
Upper right chest pain
Leucopenia   *- reduction of white blood cells*
Target Organ - Liver
Ballooning of hepatocytes
Coagulation necrosis
Cytoplasm has a ground-glass appearance
Lymphocytes respond to viral antigens
Regeneration on recovery complete

Course of Disease:
    Ingestion
    Multiplication of virus in intestinal epithelium
    Viremia
    Via portal system to liver

Complications: Cirrhosis

Diagnosis:
    Liver biopsy
    Serum enzyme test - serum transaminase increased
    Bilirubin increased
    Monitor → Liver functions tests

Serology - Immunoclectron microscopy
         ELISA

Treatment:
    Symptomatic - Bed rest
             Nutritious diet/vitamins
             No exercise
             No alcohol
    Visitors - gamma globulin
    Highly contagious-enteric isolation
         Use of disposable maximized
             (incinerate)
         Urine/fecal matter treated with phenolic compounds
         Organism resistant to boiling for 20-30 minutes
             180°F for over an hour

Epidemiology:
    Over 30,000 cases/year
    Mostly autumn/winter
    Control via isolation of carriers problem asymptomatic
        cases

No treatment
lots of
VITAMINS

NAME OF DISEASE: Unnamed (Hepatitis E disease)

Causative Organism: Hepatitis E Virus (HEV)

Characteristics of Organism:
    ss RNA
    Non-enveloped

Clinical Symptoms:
    Like infectious hepatitis
    Mortality rates highest in pregnant women

    Many forms
        1. Adults -   mild disease
                         resembles infectious mononucleosis
                         frequently post-perfusion
        2. Perinatal -   exposure in vagina
                         interstitial pneumonitis
                         mononucleosis symptoms
        3. Congenital
                         hepatosplenomegaly
                         jaundice
                         capillary bleeding
                         microcephaly/hydrocephaly
                         ocular inflammation
                         thrombocytopenia purpura
                                 (reduced platelets)
                         less of site
                         retardation
                         member of TORCH group
        4. Disseminated
                         Immunological compromised
                         AIDS
                         leukemia
                         transplant patients
                         corticosteroid therapy
                         large doses of transfusional blood
                         pneumonitis
                         hepatitis
                         myocarditis

*like Hep A
But NOT as
severe*

*Is quite
serious*

thyroiditis
meningoencephalitis
hemolytic anemia
thrombocytopenia

Diagnosis:
    Cytology -   observe inclusions
                cytomegaly (saliva, urine, sputum)
    Culture -   human embryonic fibroblasts
                human adenoid cells
                human kidney cells
    Serology -   immuno - fluorescence
                indirect hemagglutination
                complement - fixation

Treatment: Gancyilovir
            Foscarnet

Epidemiology
    1% of neonatal deaths
    4,000 deaths/year
    6,000 children with future problems/year
    antibody levels increase in adult population to a maximum
        of about 81% in the over 35-year old age group

NAME OF DISEASE: Infectious mononucleosis
OTHER NAME(S):   Mono, Kissing disease, glandular fever

Causative Organism: Epstein-Barr Virus (EBV)

Characteristics of Organism:
     Herpetovirus
     dsDNA virus - linear genome
     Enveloped
     Cubic - 162 capsomeres

Portal of Entry: Oro-pharyngeal route

Clinical Symptoms:
     Incubation - 30 to 50 days
     Due to B-cell proliferation and immune response
     Gray-white exudate in throat
     Sore throat
     Skin
     Lymphadenopathy - symmetrical, tender
                           nodes soft
     Fluctuation temperature - 103°-104°F/chills
     Sweating
     Fatigue
     Anorexia
     Lymphocytosis
     Hepatosplenomegaly

Course of Disease:
     Oropharynx to parotid gland
     Source of viremia
     Virus in blood react with B-cells
     Creating atypical lymphocytes
     T_k (cytotoxic), T_s (suppressor) cells
     Attacking plasma cells
     Virus continues to reside in B-cells
     Life long infection

Handwritten notes in margin: Associated w/ cancer; exchange of saliva; Must Monitor the spleen; last 2 weeks

Complications:
    Splenic rupture
    Facial palsies
    Encephalitis
    Hemolytic anemia
    Thrombocytopenia
    Heart defects
    Liver malfunction

Diagnosis:
    Hematology -   Blood smear
                    Downey cells - cells with granular
                        cytoplasm and vacuoles
    Differential - Lymphocytosis
                    Neutropenia
                    Atypical lymphocytes - lobated nuclei,
                        basophilic cytoplasms, vacuoles
    Serology -   Paul - Bunnel
                    Heterophilic antibody
                    Fluorescent Antibody Test for IgM
    Skin Test -   Monospot

Treatment: Symptomatic

Epidemiology:
    Peak incidence in 18-25 year olds
    Adult population 90% infected
                    20% virus in saliva
    100,000+ cases a year
    EBV also associated with Fatigue Syndrome and Burkitts
        lymphoma - a type of cancer

VIRAL DISEASES

VIA

BLOOD AND BODY FLUIDS

Serum hepatitis
Hepatitis C
Un-named (Hepatitis D)
Cytomegalovirus inclusion disease
AIDS

NAME OF DISEASE: Serum hepatitis
OTHER NAME(S):   Viral Hepatitis B, Homologous serum, Jaundice, Post-vaccinal hepatitis, Long-incubation hepatitis, Transfusion jaundice

Causative Organism: Hepatitis B Virus (HBV)

Characteristics of Organism:
    Unclassified
    DNA virus, circular genome
        part double-stranded, part single-stranded
    Dane particle - complete virion
        42 nanometers
        cubic
        dimer capsid
            outer protein - hepatitis B
            surface antigen (HBsAg)
            also called Australian antigen
            forms 20 nanometer spherical particle
            filamentous form -
            inner protein - hepatitis B
            core antigen (HBcAg)
    Juarg particle
        23-27 nanometers
        in liver parenchymal cells appears to be viral
            core

Portal of Entry:
        Intravenous needles
        Blood
        Contaminated instruments
        Sexually
        Tattooing

Clinical Symptoms:
    Incubation - 60-160 days
    Symptoms similar to hepatitis A
        (less likely fever, headache)
    Symptoms onset less abrupt

long incubation period [handwritten note]

Diagnosis: Liver enzyme test - Serum transaminase increased

Serology -   HbsAg and HbcAg in blood
Immunoelectrophoresis
Fluorescent antibody
Counter electrophoresis
Radio-immunoprecipitation
Gel-immunodiffusion

Treatment: Symptomatic -   similar to infectious hepatitis
blood/body fluid isolation
visitors - gamma globulin

Bed Rest
Monitor liver

Epidemiology:
Year round/mildly contagious
25,000 or more cases/year - 4,000-5,000 deaths
Incidence increasing
Problem in blood banking
Vaccine introduced in 1981
Newest version - recombinant DNA essential
1988/89 over 12,000 health care workers got
hepatitis with about 300 deaths

Vaccine - Boosters
3 Doses.

47

NAME OF DISEASE: Hepatitis C
OTHER NAME(S):   NANB Hepatitis, Not A-Not B Hepatitis

Causative Agent - Hepatitis C Virus (HVC)

Characteristics of Organism:
        RNA Virus
        About 27 nanometers
        Enveloped

Portal of Entry: Transfusion - 80% of cases

Clinical Symptoms:
        Incubation - 7-9 weeks
        Similar serum hepatitis

Positive RNA

No jaundice

NAME OF DISEASE: Un-named (Hepatitis D disease)

Causative Agent: Hepatitis D Virus (HDV)   *Delta Agent*

Characteristics of Organism:
    Defective particle - piggy-backs into host cell with
        hepatitis B
            ssRNA
            HB_sAg present
            36 nanometers
            enveloped

Clinical Symptoms:
    Super infection with HBV
    Increased liver damage
    Arthritis
    Rash
    Rare-arterial inflammation

Epidemiology:
    Remains infective in dried blood or serum for months at
        room temperature
    Not affected by heat up to 60°C
    Disinfectants - glutaraldehyde, iodine, chlorine

makes B much worse

IV drug transmitted

49

NAME OF DISEASE: Cytomegalovirus inclusion disease
OTHER NAME(S):   CID, generalized salivary gland disease

Causative Agent: Cytomegalovirus (CMV)

Characteristics of Organism:
   Heypetovirus
   dsDNA, linear genome
   65-120 nanometers
   Enveloped cubic - 162 capsomeres
   Latent infection
   Cytopathic effect -cytomegaly of host cell
      inclusions - lipshutz bodies
      (owl-eye)
      large, intranuclear
      acidophilic (eosinophilic)
      granules (maybe intracytoplasmic as
       well) variable in shape, nucleus
       enlarged, chromatin marginated

Portal of Entry: Oral route - salivary secretions
      Congenital
      Perinatal
      Venereal
      Respiratory
      Transfusional
      Transplantational
  (target/severity determined by portal of entry)

NAME OF DISEASE: AIDS
OTHER NAME(S):   Acquired immune deficiency syndrome

Causative Organism: HIV I and II
    (Human immuno deficiency virus)
    previously called HTLV-III
    and LAV - lymphadenopathy virus

Characteristics of Organism
    Retrovirus
    ssRNA virus/enveloped
    uses reverse transcriptase
    major CPE - transformation
    Sensitive to heat/disinfectant

Portal of Entry:
    Contact with body fluids
    In particular blood/semen

Clinical Symptoms:
    Initially a cluster of symptoms
        Kaposi's sarcoma
        Pneumocystosis pneumonia
        Weight loss
        Swollen lymph nodes
        Loss of immunity

Clinical definition now
    Opportunistic infections
        (particularly, Mycobacterium)
    Unusual cancers
        Chronically swollen lymph nodes
        Weight loss
        Diarrhea
        Neurological disorders

Virus infects dendritic cells, bone marrow, blood, macrophages - multiplies without destroying cells.

Destroys T-4 cells, monocytes, B-lymphocytes

51

Diagnosis:
      ELISA test
      Patient History
      LAT (latex agglutination test) **99% accurate**
      Western blot - more accurate

Treatment:
      Symptomatic for infections

VIRAL DISEASES
VIA
DIRECT CONTACT

Herpes
Genital Herpes
Venereal Warts

NAME OF DISEASE: Herpes

OTHER NAME(S):   Fever blisters, cold sores, herpes labialism, gingiva-stomatitis (around mouth) eczema hetpeticum (skin), herpetic keratitis (eyes), herpetic gladiotorum (body)

Causative Organism: Herpes simplex virus - Type I (HSV-1) also called Herpes virus homimus - Type 1 (HVH-1)

Characteristics of Organism:
    Herpetovirus
    ds DNA - linear genome
    100 nanometers
    cubic - 162 capsomere
    enveloped-prominent spikes
    Cell-to-Cell transfer - cell fusion factors
    Cytopathic effect -   giant cells
        inclusion-lipshutz bodies-
        well-defined variable
        shaped, acidophilic
        (eosinophilic)inclusions
    Relatively sensitive to environmental factors

Portal of Entry:
    Direct Contact with mucous membrane

Clinical Symptoms:
    Virus effects basal cells and epithelial cells
    Localized edema
    Lysis of cells
    Cell fusion
    Degeneration of tissue
    Ballooning causing formation of vesicles
    Incubation - 2 to 14 days
    Herpetic keratitis (ocular herpes) - unilateral conjunctivitis
    opaque corneal lesions, vesicles on lid
    Route ocular branch of trigeminal, local adenopathy

Herpetic whitlow - first it tingles - then red, swollen,
          painful, itchy
          damaged skin
          may form red streak up a arm
Herpetic gingivostomatitis -
          mostly seen in infants
          gums red/swollen
          ulcers in mouth
          dysphagia
          pharyngitis

In pap smear -   observe enlarge, multinucleated cells
                intranuclear inclusions
Encephalitis -   personality change
                convulsions
                seizures

General symptoms:
        tingling/itching
        vesicles erupt on erythromatous
        base
        rupture
        ulcerate
        yellowish crust
        Resolution - 10-21 days
        Fever may or may not be present

Complication:
        life-long infection
        Re-eruption - predispositions-
          stress
          trauma
          ultraviolet light
          hormones
          metabolic changes

Diagnosis:
        Microscopic -   Corneal scrapings
                    Spinal fluid
                    Vesicular Fluid
                    All examined for lipshutz bodies

55

Cultural -   Human embryonic lung fibroblasts
chicken embryo

Serology -   Fluorescent - antibody
Viral neutralization
Complement - fixation
Monoclonal antibodies
Fluorescent dyes
    enzymes

Treatment:
Stoxil (Idoxuridine)
Herpetic Keratitis - trifluridine
Encephalitis/neonatal - adenine arabinoside (ARA-A)
                    vidarabine (Vira-A)

Epidemiology:
Encephalitis -   untreated - 70% fatalities
treated - 10% will lead normal lives

NAME OF DISEASE: Genital Herpes

Causative Organism: Herpes simplex - Type II (HSV II)

Characteristics of Organism:
      See Herpes
      Type II - more heat sensitive
              forms larger pox on chick embryo
              more virulent
              more resistant to drugs

Portal of Entry:
      Venereal

Clinical Symptoms:
      Pain and itching
      Eruption of thin walled vesicles
      on erythematous elevated base
      Highly infectious
      Rupture
      Scab
      Heal
      Frequently Fever
      Muscle aches - leg, particular
      Dysuria
      Regional lymphadenopathy

Complication:
    Neonatal encephalitis - picked up while passage through
    vaginal canal
    Part of TORCH group
    Active infection in female at delivery
      indication - caesarian section
    Life long, infection virus resides in sacral root ganglion

Diagnosis:
    See Herpes

Treatment:
    Acyclovir (Zovirax)
    Neonate - see herpes

NAME OF DISEASE: Venereal warts

Causative Organism: Human papilloma virus (HPV)

Characteristics of Organism:
    Papovavirus
    ds DNA - Closed circle genome
    Slow growing in host cell nucleus
    Non-enveloped
    45-55 nanometers - 72 capsomeres

Portal of Entry:
    Venereal

Clinical Symptoms:
    Incubation -   dermal - 1 month
                    venereal up to 8 months
    painless elevated, rough, lesions - fingers
    deep, painful - soles of feet
    smooth, flat, skin-colored - face/trunk
    Fusion of many small flat bumps
    giant cauliflower mass called condylomata acuminata
    Laryngeal lesions, large and benign

    In Dermis - distinct boundary above
    basement membrane between dermis-epidermis

        Genital lesions - possibly malignant

Diagnosis:
    Clinical picture
    Serology -   ELISA
                 Immunofluorescent Antibody
Treatment:
    Cryotherapy
    Electrodesiccation
    Acid burning
    Injection of Interferon
    Lasers - care by physician
                aerosolic virus - contagious

[handwritten margin notes: DNA grow slower; slow growing]

58

VIRAL DISEASE

VIA

ANIMAL BITES

Rabies - fury

NAME OF DISEASE: Rabies
OTHER NAME(S): Hydrophobia

Causative Organism: Rabies virus

Characteristics of Organism:
    Rhabdovirus
    ss RNA
    Enveloped/helical
    75 x 180 nanometers
    Bullet-shaped
    Cytopathic Effect -
            Inclusion bodies
            Negri - dark oval, cytoplasmic, acidophilic
            inclusions in neurons

Portal of Entry: Bite of Animal
                    In reality saliva is infectious
                    Transmitted via respiratory route
                    Also inhalation of rabid bat feces

Saliva not bite, the deeper the bite the more severe

Clinical Symptoms:
    Incubation - 6 days to 12 months
                  depending on location and severity of bite and
                  amount of virus introduced
    Initially -   low grade fever (100-102°F)
                  headache
                  restlessness
                  tingling, burning, coldness at bite site
                  loose cough
    Followed -   personality change
                  aggressive/agitated
                  excessive salivation, perspiration
                  sensitive to noise
                  tachycardia
                  shallow respiration
                  pupillary dilation
                  fever rises
                  muscle spasms in throat
                  aerophobia

heart speed up

60

Final stage - paralysis
               death

Course of Disease:
     Virus introduced by bite
     Via blood to muscle
     Virus multiplies
     Spreads to nerves (degeneration/demyelination of neurons)
     To brain via nerves

Diagnosis:
        Animal -   Observe ten days
                   Destroy, brain sections - observe negri
                      bodies (not necessary if no symptoms)
                   Serology -   Seller's antibody test
                                Fluorescent Antibody test
                                Seller's stain technique
                                (hippocampal cells)

        Patient -   Clinical picture
                   Animal bite
                   Any wild animal bite treated as rabid
                   (if not captured)

Treatment:
        Wound -   Soap/water
                   Iodine
                   Alcohol
                   Fuming Nitric Acid
                   Topical ARS (antirabies serum - available
                       in field first aid kits)

Follow-up - Injectable Rabies antisera
                   (passive immunity)
                   either PRS or HRIG
                   Rabies vaccine - active immunity
                   use HDCV - Human diploid cell
                   vaccine (Merieux)

Epidemiology:
    Two forms in animals
        Furious - violent
                    wide-eyed
                    drools
                    shaking of head
                    attacks
        Dumb -   lethargic
                    cowardly
                    cough (highly infectious-
                        do not approach)

Vaccine -   Original by Pasteur
        Serial passage in rabbit brains

        For dogs and cats today - use avianized or
            duck embryo vaccine (DEV)
        Two forms - HEP - high egg passage
            for adults
            LEP - low egg passage for puppies

VIRAL DISEASES

VIA

INSECT BITES

Viral Encephalitis
Yellow fever
Dengue
Colorado Tick Fever
West Nile Fever
Russian Spring-Summer Encephalitis
Japanese B Encephalitis
Lassa Fever

NAME OF DISEASE: Viral Encephalitis
Causative Organism: various types of Group A arbovirus

Characteristics of Organism:
        Togavirus
            Subdivision alpharvirus
    ssRNA
    Cubical/enveloped
    50 - 70 nanometers / 32 capsomeres
    Hemagglutinin positive
    Cultured in fertile eggs and Hela cells

Portal of Entry:
    Break in Skin
        Vector Mosquito - Aedes
                    Culex
                    Anopheles
                    Culiesta
    Reservoir - rodents, birds, horses
    Zoonosis - a disease of animals
            Man incidental host

Clinical Symptoms:
    Incubation - 1 day-to-several weeks
    General description inflammation of brain
        Rapid onset of symptoms
        Chills/fever (high)
        Headache
        Cyanosis
        Vomiting
        Disorientation/drowsiness
        Muscular twitching

    Encephlistic state - follows
        amnesia
        convulsions/tremor
        paralysis
        coma
        notable increase intercranial pressure

Types
>Eastern Equine Encephalitis - EEE
>>Most severe - mortality 70-80%
>>Necrotizing infection/permanent damage
>>kills in days
>>Occurrence in rainier parts of late summer
>>Neutrophilic infiltration of brain
>>Resembles pyogenic infection
>>Vasculitis/thromboses
>>Areas of necrosis resembles microabcesses
>>Perivascular cuffing
>Western Equine Encephalitis (WEE)
>>Usually effects younger children
>>Mortality less then 10%
>>About 100 cases/year
>>More lymphocytic infiltration then neutrophilic
>Venezuelan Equine Encephalitis (VEE)
>>Resembles flu
>>Mild infection
>California Encephalitis (CE)
>>"Lacrosse" strain
>>Mild disease
>>Headache, nausea, fever
>>Mostly children - rural regions
>St. Louis encephalitis - (SLE)
>>Most commonly reported form
>>200$^+$ cases/year
>>Most severe in elderly - other symptoms
>>Headache/delirium, fever
>>Muscle rigidity
>>Muscle tremor
>>Anorexia
>>Myalgia
>>Urinary tract infection
>>Spinal fluid - increased opening pressure
>>pleocytosis

Course of Disease:
      Through skin to lymph nodes
      Virus multiples in blood
      Viremia
      Brain and CNS

Diagnosis:
      Viral Isolation
            Culture - Hela cells - marked cytopathic effect
            Serology - Hemagglutination - chicken/geese blood
                      Neutralization test

Treatment:
      Symptomatic

Epidemiology:
      Vaccine for horses - formalin - inactivated
                    grown in chicken embryo
      Risk group -   workers with or around horses
      Prevention -   immunization of horses
                    quarantine
                    insect control

NAME OF DISEASE: Yellow Fever
Causative Organism: Yellow Fever Virus
                      Group B arbovirus

Characteristics of Organism:
   Togavirus
   subdivision - flavivirus
   ssRNA
   cubical/enveloped
   56-62 nanometers /32 capsomeres
   Cultured -   Maintained minced chicken embryo
                     Human appendix tissue culture
                     Human conjunctival tissue
                     Cytopathic effect - Inclusion bodies
                     Councilman bodies - intense
                     acidophilic (eosinophilic) oval
                     bodies, in necrotic parenchymal cells
                     which have lost nuclei

Portal of Entry:
   Break in skin
      Vector -   <u>Aedes</u> <u>aegypti</u>
                <u>Haemogogus</u>
     Reservoir - monkeys (don't get disease)

Clinical Symptoms:
   Incubation 3-6 days
   Two stages

      1.   Fever/chills
           Headache
           Myalgia
           Lasts 3-4 days

      2.   Gastro - intestinal symptoms
           Bloody stools
           Hemoptysis
           Black
           Vomitus
           Slow pulse

Leukopenia
Hypotension
Hepatic failure -   fatty infiltration
Bile stained
Midzonal necrosis
jaundice
Albuminuria
Renal failure -   Coagulative necrosis
of proximal tubules
fat in tublar
epithelium
hemorrhagic
hematuria

Bleeding diathesis
Heals with Sequelae

Mortality - untreated about 40%
treated about 5%

Course of Disease:
Mosquito ingests blood form victim with yellow fever
9-10 days incubation in mosquito
via mosquito's saliva to next victim
To lymph nodes - virus multiplies
Viremia
To liver, spleen, kidney, heart

Diagnosis:
Histology -   Liver biopsy

Serology -   Neutralization test
complement fixation

Treatment:
Symptomatic/Supportive
Blood transfusion convalescent (hyper-immune) serum

Epidemiology:
   Vaccines - two types
      1.   Subcutaneous - 17D strain virus
           Grown in chicken embryo

      2.   Scarification - dakar strain
           cultured in mouse brain

NAME OF DISEASE: Dengue
OTHER NAME (S):   Breakbone Fever, Eland Fever,
                        Saddleback fever
Causative Organism: Dengue virus
                        (Group B Arbovirus)

Characteristics of Organism:
    Togavirus
        subdivision - Flavivirus
        ssRNA
        17-25 nanometers / enveloped
        cubical /32 capsomere
        difficult to culture
        four antigenic types

Portal of Entry:
    Break in skin
        vector - <u>Aedes</u> <u>aegypti</u>
                 <u>Aedes</u> <u>albopictus</u>
        Reservoir - monkey

Clinical Symptoms:
    Incubation - 5 to 8 days
    Two diseases
        1.   Dengue -   sharp rise in temperature
                          Prostration
                          Extreme pain in limbs
                          Photophobia
                          Alterration in taste
                          Recovery ~5 to 6 days

        2.   Dengue Hemorraghic Fever (DHF)
                          Immunological response
                          Two antigenic types infect sequentially
                          Rash - face and extremities
                          Severe vomiting
                          High fever
                          Intestinal hemorrhage
                          Thrombocytopenia
                          Neurological disturbances

Diagnosis:
   Serology - complement - fixation

Treatment:
   Symptomatic

Epidemiology:
   Vaccine for antigenic type II
            live, attenuated vaccine

71

NAME OF DISEASE: Colorado Tick Fever
OTHER NAME(S):   Saddleback Fever

Causative Organism: Colorado Tick Fever Virus

Characteristics of Organism:
    Bunyavirus
    ss RNA
    20 nanometer
    Helical/enveloped
    Replicates in cytoplasm - buds via golgi

Portal of Entry:
    Break in skin
        Vector - tick (Dermacentor)

Clinical Symptoms:
    Incubation - 3 to 6 days
    Chills/Fever (104°F)
    Headache
    Severe muscular pain
    Joint pain
    Eyepain
    Nausea/vomiting
    Leukopenia
    Thrombocytopenia

Complications:
    Meningoencephalitis
    Orchitis

Diagnosis:
    Serology -   Fluorescent - antibody
            Complement - Fixation

Treatment:
    Symptomatic

Epidemiology:
    Vaccine -   grown fertile hen's egg
    Endemic to Colorado - about 150+ cases per year.

73

NAME OF DISEASE: West Nile Fever
Causative Organism: West Nile Fever Virus
                              (Group B arbovirus)

Characteristics of Organism:
     Togavirus
          subdivision - Flaviviurs
          20-40 nanometers /32 capsomeres
          ss RNA
          cubical/enveloped
          Cultured -   swiss mice brain
                            fertile hen's eggs

Portal of Entry:
     Break in skin
     Vector mosquito

Clinical Symptoms:
     fever
     lymphadenopathy
     rash
     headache
     pain in chest and back
     convalescence slow

Diagnosis:
     Serology -   Fluorescein - labelled antibody

Treatment:
     Symptomatic

NAME OF DISEASE: Russian Spring-Summer Encephalitis
OTHER NAME(S):   Wood cutters encephalitis,
Forest-spring encephalitis, tick borne encephalitis, vernoestival encephalitis

Causative Organism: Russian Spring-Summer Encephalitis Virus
(Group B arbovirus)

Characteristics of Organism:
  Togavirus
      subdivision - Flavivurus
      20 nanometers /32 capsomere
      ss RNA
      cubical/enveloped

Portal of Entry:
      Break in skin
      vector - tick (Ixodes)

Clinical Symptoms:
      Incubation - 8 to 18 days
          fever
          headache
          nausea/vomiting
          vertigo
          cervical pain
          paralysis possible - 2 or 3 days
          virus in CSF
          duration - 2 to 10 days

Complications:
      Serology - complement - fixation

Treatment:
      Symptomatic

Epidemiology:
      2 vaccines -   One cultured in mouse brain tissue
                    Another cultured in fertile hen's egg

NAME OF DISEASE: Japanese B encephalitis
OTHER NAME(S):   B encephalitis, summer encephalitis

Causative Organism: Japanese B encephalitis virus
                                  (Group B arbovirus)

Characteristics of Organism:
        Togavirus
                subdivision - flavivirus
                ss RNA
                cubical /32 capsomere
                20-30 nanometers
                enveloped
                cultured -   minced chicken embryo brain
                                   fertile hen's egg's
                                   Hela cells

Portal of Entry:
    Break in skin
        vector -   culex
        reservoir -   rodent
                        mosquito over winter

Clinical Symptoms:
    Incubation - 6 to 8 days
        fever
        headache/delirium
        paralysis
        mental/personality change
        coma

Diagnosis:
    Serology -   complement fixation
                        neutralization

Treatment:
   Three vaccines
1. Formaldehyde inactivate virus grown in mouse brain
2. Virus grown in chicken embryo and stabilized via lyophilization
3. Live attenuated virus, grown in hamster kidney tissue - least effective.

NAME OF DISEASE: Lassa Fever
OTHER NAME(S):   Lassa hemorrhagic fever

Causative Organisms: Lassa Fever Virus

Characteristics of Organism:
    Arenavirus
    Possibly helical
    ss RNA
    Enveloped
    150 - 175 nanometers
    Sandy granules viewed under electron microscopy

Portal of Entry:
    Respiratory Route
    Rodent parasites-vectors

Clinical Symptoms:
    Incubation 2 to 4 days (average)
    Abrupt onset
    Fever
    Pharyngitis
    Lymphadenopathy
    Patchy hemorrhagic lesions on throat
        (bleeding obstructs breathing)
    Profuse internal hemorrhaging
    Erythrocytopenia
    Most severe if mucous membranes involved

Complications:
    Hepatitis
    Myocarditis
    Secondary bacteria infections

Diagnosis:
    Serology

Treatment:
    Symptomatic

Epidemiology:
   Other hemorrhagic fevers

Omsk Hemorrhagic Fever -   high fever
hemorrhage-mucous membrane
pneumonitis
pulmonary hemorrhage/edema
Reservoir - small rodents
                domesticated
                     animals

Crimean Hemorrhagic Fever -   Like OHF

Bolivian Hemorrhagic Fever -   Lymph/bone
Marrow involvement
Vascular damage
Bleed/shock
CNS involved

Korean Hemorrhagic Fever - Diapedes of RBC's
Loss of blood
Shock
Renal Damage
Liver/spleen
Mononuclear cell infiltrate
Source - saliva
Urine of rodents

Argentinean Hemorrhagic Fever -
Like Korean
Source airborne or food
Reservoir-rodents

Chibunjunga Hemorrhagic Fever -
Fever
Muscular/joint pain
Myocarditis
Hematemesis
Melena
Shock

Man - reservoir

Mortality in all -   30 to 70%

Control by controlling -   rodents

                                           animals
                                           excreta
                                           airborne aersolic
                                           particles

Other hemorrhagic fevers include - Rift Valley Fever
                                                      Indian hemorrhagic Fever
                                                       Ebola Fever

SLOW VIRUS

Marburg Disease
Jacob - Crutzfeld Disease
Ebola Fever

NAME OF DISEASE: Marburg Disease
OTHER NAME(S):   Green Monkey Disease

Causative Organism: Marburg Virus

Characteristics of Organism:
      Filovirus
      RNA Virus
      Helical Symmetry
      130 - 400 nanometers

Portal of Entry:
      Blood of monkeys?

Clinical Symptoms:
      Severe sore throat
      Fever
      Recovery
      Relapse
      Maculo papular rash - face, trunk, extremities
      Red exanthemas - hard/soft palate
      Bleeding gums/from nose
      Generalized bleeding - gastro -intestinal
      Edema of brain
      Kidney/liver - cell death
      Mortality - high

Diagnosis:
      Serology

Treatment:
      Symptomatic

NAME OF DISEASE: Jacob Crutzfeld Disease

Causative Organism: Unidentified

Portal of Entry:
Unclear
Patient to neurosurgeon
(Contaminated instruments)
Corneal Transplants

Clinical Symptoms:
Spongioform degeneration of cerebral cortex
No fever/no inflammation

Treatment:
Symptomatic

NAME OF DISEASE: Ebola Fever
OTHER NAME(S):   Ebola Viral Disease

Causative Organism: Ebola Virus

Characteristics of Organism:
        Filovirus
        RNA
        Helical
        Fishbone - shaped
        130-400 nanometers

Portal of Entry:
    Unproven
    Close/prolonged contact with infected person
    Needles/syringes

Clinical Symptoms:
    See Marburg's

Treatment:
    Symptomatic

MYCOPLASMAL DISEASE

Primary Atypical Pneumonia
Non - specific Urethritis

- small known
organism
Independent

NAME OF DISEASE: Primary Atypical Pneumonia
OTHER NAME(S):   Eaton's agent pneumonia, mycoplasmal
pneumonia

Causative Organism: <u>Mycoplasma pneumonia</u>

Characteristics of Organism:
    Smallest free-living
    organism
    Non-cell wall/plastic
    0.2 micrometers in size
    Plemorophic
    Requires high levels of
    sterol in media - Brain -
    Heart *(high cholesreial)*
    Infusion with horse
    serum *- Rich in Cholesterial*

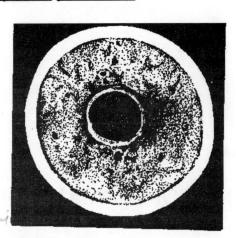

Fried egg appearance of
mycoplasmal colony

Portal of Entry:
    Respiratory via droplet
      spray
    Direct - contaminated fomites

Clinical Symptoms:
    Incubation - 1 to 3 weeks
    Children more severe than adults
        Children -   cough
                    rales (abnormal rattling - bubbling)
                    fever (higher 103°F)/chills
        Adults -   in addition - headache, sore throat
        Duration -   7 to 10 days or even 4 to 6 weeks
    Cough begins as non-productive
    Followed by watery or mucus sputum
    Pleurisy
    Rhinorrhea
        Internal -   patchy interstitial pneumonia
                    swollen alveolar linings
                        (reduced alveolar space)
                    Bronchial wall thickening-edema

Procaryotic

WALKING Pneumonia

No shape Flexibility

motility visabile under micro

granular

86

Intraluminal exudates contain
  neutrophils
  epithelial cells
  proteinaceous liquid
Tissue infiltrated - first by
  lymphocytes
  Then - neutrophils
  macrophages

Epithehal damage
Ciliostasis

Complications:
  Encephalitis
  Polyneuritis
  Aseptic meningitis
  Acute psychosis
  Guillane - Barre Syndrome

Diagnosis:

Serology -   Cold Agglutination Screening Test (CAST)
                  Occurs at 4°C not 37°C
                  Completion Fixation test
                  Fluorescent Antibody Test
                  DNA probe

Cultural -   Yeast extract, penicillin, serum, thallium
                  acetate (prevent contamination)
                  slow growing
                  Colonies 10 - 200 mm.

                  On Guinea pig-blood - alpha hemolysis -
                    distinguishes from other mycoplasma

                  Mycoplasmal broth - phenol red-acid
                    fermentation

Stain -   Methylene blue/Azure II using gentle heat

Treatment:
      Erythromycin
      Tetracycline

Epidemiology:
      Vaccine used in military
      500,000 cases per year
      In top ten causes of death

NOTES:

NAME OF DISEASE: Non-specific urethritis
OTHER NAME(S): Non-gonoccal urethritis, NGU, NSU

Causative Organism: <u>Ureaplasm</u> <u>Urealyticum</u>
also called T-strain mycoplasma

Breaks urea (handwritten)

Characteristics of Organism:
See Mycoplasma pneumonia

Notable feature - hydrolyses urea

Portal of Entry:
Transmitted sexually

Clinical Symptoms:
Similar to gonorrhea

Complications:
Pelvic Inflammatory Disease

Diagnosis:
See Primary Atypical Pneumonia

Treatment:
Tetracycline
Tetracycline - resistant use erythromycin

OR Spectinomycin (handwritten)

Epidemiology - Implicated
Low birth weight
Premature birth
Spontaneous abortion
Infertility

IMPACTS FETUS. Moves into cervix (handwritten)

89

TREATMENT : TETRACYCLINE

RICKETTSIAL DISEASES

Endemic → Epidemic Typhus
Epidemic Typhus
Rockey Mountain Spotted Fever
Boutoneuse Fever
North Queensland Tick Fever
Siberian Tick Bite Typhus
Tsutsugamushi Fever
Rickettsialpox
Trench Fever
Q-Fever

NOTES:

NAME OF DISEASE: Epidemic typhus *means lazy*
OTHER NAME(S): Classic typhus, European typhus, Old-World typhus, Jail fever, War Fever, Famine Fever, Louse-Borne typhus (7)

Causative Organism: *class/Genus* Rickettsia prowazekii

Characteristics of Organism:
    Obligate Intracellular parasite - leaky membranes lose metabolites
    Coccobacillus - 0.3-0.5 micrometers by 0.3 micrometers
    Staining properties - Gram - Negative (pink)
                          Giesnsa - blue to purple
                          Machiavelle's - red
                          Gimenez - red *-magenta*
    Multiplies in host's endothelial cells
    Non-motile
    Cultured in yolk sac of fertilized hen's eggs

Portal of Entry:
    Break in skin
    Vector - Human body louse - Pediculus humanus*
    also called - Pediculus corporis
    rarely - Pediculus capitis
    *Prefers environment between 20-30∘C
    Also - Respiratory via dried louse feces
    Conjunctival via rubbing

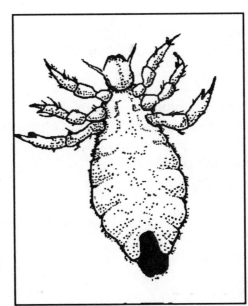

Pediculous corporis

reside in clothing Blood suckers defecates

Clinical Symptoms:
    Incubation - 5 to 21 days, average 10-14 days
    Rapid rise in temperature 103-104∘F

Chills, depression, weakness
Unremitting, severe, frontal headache
Pain in limbs
4th - 7th day -   rash appears
                First on palms and soles
                Rash starts pink to purple to brownish red
                Rash begins macular and becomes maculopapular
Irregular heart beat/low blood pressure
Cough
Lethargy
Enlarged spleen
Oliguria
Damage blood vessels - growth in endothelium
       endothehal perforation
       thrombosis
       hemorrhage
       hemoconcentration
Stupor/Delirium
Shock/Death
Untreated -   10% in children
             40-60% in adults over 50

Course of Disease:
    Louse feeds on host's blood
    Defecates -   feces contains rickettsia, can survive in feces
               for up to 3 months
    Saliva irritates edges of wound
    Scratch and self inoculate

Complications:
    Parotitis
    Suppurative otitis media
    Mastoiditis
    Gangrene of extremities
    Bronchitis
    Encephalitis

Lymph

Diagnosis:

Serological - Weil-Felix Test - Four-Fold
increase acute versus convalescent serum
Serum
Agglutinates - <u>P. vulgaris</u> OX-19-strongly
<u>P. vulgaris</u> OX-2-weakly
Complement - Fixation Test
Indirect Fluorescent Antibody Test

Typhus group
Spotted fever Group
OXK -

Treatment:

Tetracycline
Chloramphenicol
Sulfa drugs - contra-indicated because increases severity
of disease

LAST RESORT
Not Recommended

Control of Disease:

Delousing with DDT or other insecticide
Proper hygiene and bathing
Insecticidal powders
Removing clothes - temperature drops, lice leave
Vaccine - Cox - Formalin-killed vaccine (also attenuated
vaccine)
(useful only in epidemics)

Other:

Brill's Disease also called Brill-Zinsser Disease, Sporadic
typhus, Recrudescent typhus relapse
without exposure to lice 30-40 years later
after initial infection
Predisposition - stress
lowered immunity
Symptoms milder, no rash
Last 2 weeks rather than 3-5 weeks
Fever intermittent

93

NAME OF DISEASE: Endemic typhus
OTHER NAME(S): Murine typhus, Flea-borne typhus, New-World typhus, urban typhus, shop typhus, Toulon typhus, Manchurian typhus, Red Fever (Congo), Tarbadillo (American Southwest)

Causative Organism: <u>Rickettsia</u> <u>typhi</u>
also called <u>Rickettsia</u> <u>mooseri</u>

Characteristics of Organism:
See epidemic typhus

Portal of Entry:
Break in skin
Vector-rat flea
(<u>Xenopsyllus</u>)
Reservoir rats

Clinical Symptoms:

Common 1 week

Incubation - 6-14 days
Milder than epidemic typhus
Mortality less than 3%

Rat Flea – murine typhus and plague

Differences from Epidemic typhus
hacking cough
irregular eruption of rash *(Rose colored)*
nausea/vomiting
rash - frequently concentrated on shoulders and back as in tarbadillo

Course of Disease:
Rat to rat via flea
Man incidental host
Rickettsia transmitted transovarially to offspring

Diagnosis:

Serology -	Weil-Felix - same as <u>R. prowazekii</u>
	complement - fixation
Cytology -	Guinea Pig scrotal cells
	Observation intracytoplasmic Mooseri
	Bodies

Treatment: Same as Epidemic typhus

Control of Disease:
 Rat control
 Garbage collection
 Vaccination of laboratory workers
 75-100 cases per year compared to 3000-5000 cases per year in 1930's and 1940's

NAME OF DISEASE: Rocky Mountain Spotted Fever
OTHER NAME(S): American Spotted Fever, Tick Fever

Causative Organism: <u>Rickettsia</u> <u>rickettsiae</u>

Characteristics of Organism:
See Epidemic typhus

Portal of Entry:
Break in skin
Vector -

hard Ticks (<u>Dermacentor</u>, <u>Amblyomma</u>, <u>Ixodes</u>) Including wood tick, deer tick, rabbit tick, dog tick

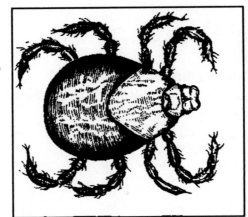

Hard Tick of Rocky
Mountain Fever

Clinical Symptoms:
Incubation 2-14 days, average 7 days
Severe headache
Pain in joints/muscles
Fever about 104ºF
Rash - begins on palms and soles, maybe forehead
  Pink to dark red or purple
  Petechial to macular to maculo-papular
  Blanches with pressure
  Some skin may become gangrenous (3 or more weeks)
  Thrombocytopenia - less than 100,000/ml
  rapid heartbeat/hypotension
  rapid respiration
  nausea/vomiting/constipation
  hepatosplenomegaly
  Tremor/deafness
  Restlessness/delirium

Muscle pain

Bleeding (nose)

96

Endothial damage -   micro-thrombi
                       micro-hemorrhage
Reduced urinary output
Ataxia

Course of Disease:
Tick feeds - 3-4 hours
Passes organisms via saliva
Rickettsia passed to tick progeny trans-ovarially

Complications:
Thromboses
Microinfacts in brain-ring hemorrhages
Renal failure
Lobar pneumonia

Diagnosis:
Serology - Weil-Felix
Four-fold increase acute versus convalescent serum
Agglutinates weakly P. vulgaris - OX-19
                                   OX-2
                                   OX-K

Fluorescent antibody test

Cytology - Guinea pig tissue
Rickettsia -   both in cytoplasm and nucleus
                 Have a floral arrangement

Hematology - leukopenia
              thrombocytopenia

Treatment:
Tetracycline - the earlier the better
Chloramphenicol - the earlier the better
Replace serum albumin, IV
Corticosteroid for toxemia
Hyperimmune serum if very early

If caught early enough administer

Control of Disease:
    Avoidance of ticks
    Proper dress in field and self examination
    Remove ticks properly
        No matches, no tweezers
        Use irritant on abdomen or oily substance to block
        spirucules so tick must pull out
    Do not crush tick - juices infective
    Vaccine - 2 varieties
        Use in high risk areas
        Expensive - cultivation cannot use penicillin to
            prevent contamination
    Over 1000 cases/year - ever increasing
    Before 1970's not known in Eastern United States
    Mostly children in rural areas in Summer/Spring
    Untreated - 20-40% mortality (higher in dark skinned races)
    Treated - 5-10% mortality

95% FATAL

Remove Tick with:
Vinegar
Nail polish remover.
Never squeeze Tick
Cold Cream
dressing
oily substance
(they will back out)

Ticks not out
in winter

98

NAME OF DISEASE: Boutoneuse Fever
OTHER NAME(S):   Mediterranean Fever, South African Tick
                   Fever, Kenya tick typhus, Indian tick bite
                   fever, Abyssinian tick fever   (5)

Ethiopia

Causative Organism: <u>Rickettsia</u> <u>conorii</u>

Characteristics of Organism:
     See Epidemic typhus

Portal off Entry: Break in skin   *lesion*
                   Vector-tick

Clinical Symptoms:
     Incubation - 1 to 2 weeks
     Eschar* (black, necrotic ulcer) at tick bite site   *redness (sore)*
     Surrounded by zone of erythema, 2-5mm
     Fever about 104°F/chills
     Headache
     Hemorrhage, maculopapular rash
     Mortality low

  * Called Tache noir

Diagnosis:
     Serology - Weil-Felix Test

     Cytology - Guinea pig scrotal cell
                Intra- and extra-nuclear rickettsia

Treatment: Tetracycline
              Chloramphenicol

NAME OF DISEASE: North Queensland Tick Fever
OTHER NAME: Queensland Tick Typhus

Causative Organism: Rickettsia australis

Characteristic of Organism:
See Epidemic typhus

Portal of Entry: Break in skin
Vector-tick

Clinical Symptoms:
Mild disease - resembles murine typhus
Zonal eschars
Mild lymphadenopathy

Treatment: Chlortetracycline   ORReo
Chlormycetin

Australia

100

NOTES:

NAME OF DISEASE: Siberian tick bite typhus
OTHER NAME: Far Eastern typhus

Causative Organism: <u>Rickettsia</u> <u>Sibirica</u>
                    also called <u>R.</u> <u>Sibericus</u>

Characteristics of Organism:
    See Epidemic typhus

Portal of Entry: Break in skin
                   Vector-tick

Clinical Symptoms:
    Incubation - 2-3 days
    Regional lymphadenitis
    Headache
    Nausea
    Fever
    Rickettsial rash
    Mortality - very low to non-existent

Treatment:
    None indicated

Flu mild disease

No Treatment

effects more Men than women

101

NAME OF DISEASE: Tsutsugamushi Fever

OTHER NAME(S):   Scrub Fever, Scrub typhus, River fever, Swamp fever, mite bite typhus, tropical typhus, Japanese typhus, dangerous bug typhus, rural fever, chigger-borne typhus

(10)

Causative Organism: <u>Rickettsia</u> <u>tsutsugamushi</u>
also called <u>Rickettsia</u> <u>orientalis</u>

Portal of Entry:
Break in skin
Vector - Trombiculid mites, chigger stage

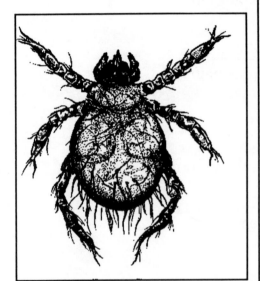

Mite (chigger) related to Tsutsugamushi Fever

Clinical Symptoms:
Incubation - 7 to 14 days, possible to 21 days
Eschar at chigger bite
Significant lymphadenopathy compared to other rickettsial diseases
Fever/chills (step-like rise in temperature)
Post-orbital pain
Nausea/vomiting
Splenomegaly
Low pulse
Red macular or maculopapular rash
Delirium/confusion
Severe cases - Necrosis of skin and lymph nodes
Mononuclear infiltration of heart and lungs

Course of Disease:
    Chigger burrows into skin
    Has blood meal
    Transmitted via saliva
    Rickettsia in chigger through nymph and adult stage
    Also passed transovarianly

Complications: Deafness
                  Mental disturbances
                  Circulatory failure
                  Encephalitis
                  Secondary bacterial pneumonia

Diagnosis:
    Serology - Weil - Felix - Four-fold increase in titre, acute
                versus convalescent serum
                agglutinates P. Vulgaris OXX-K
                Complement fixation - not a good test, 13
                different antigens

Treatment: Tetracycline
              Chloramphenicol

NAME OF DISEASE: Rickettsialpox
OTHER NAME: Russian Vesicular Rickettsiosis

Causative Organism: Rickettsia akari

Characteristics of Organism:
    See Epidemic typhus

Portal of Entry:
    Break in skin
    Vector - Urban mite (Allodermanyssus)
    Reservoir - domestic mice

Clinical Symptoms:
    Incubation - about 10 days
    Fever - 103°F, about 1 week
    Sudden chills/sweats
    Headache/Backache
    Photophobia
    Red, papular/enlarged, tender lymph nodes
    Monocytosis/Lymphocytosis
    Rash - discrete, erythromatous
          maculopapular rash
          becomes vesicular, fluid-filled
          resembles chicken-pox
          no residual scars

Diagnosis:
    Isolation of organism
    Patient's lesions to mice to fertilized hen's eggs (difficult)
    clinical picture combine with presence of eschar

Resembles Chicken Pox

TETRA Cycline

NAME OF DISEASE: Trench Fever
OTHER NAME(S):   His-Werner Disease, Shin-Bone Fever,
                      Five-Day Fever, Quintana Fever

Causative Organism:
    Rochalimea quintana
    Used to be called *Rickettsia quintana*

Characteristics of Organism:
      See Epidemic Typhus
    Notable Feature -   can be cultivated on a non-living media
                     Common media - blood agar with horse
                     erythrocytes/serum

Portal of entry:
    Break in skin
    Vector - Human body louse (*Pediculus*)
    Blood transfusions - viable a long time in blood

Clinical Symptoms:
    Fever/chilly sensation
    Headache/dizziness
    Post-orbital pain/conjunctivitis
    Nystagmus
    Back pain and in limbs
    Rapid pulse
    Splenomegaly
    Erythromatous macular/papular rash
    Recovery - 5-6 weeks

Diagnosis:
    Xenodiagnosis - Allow laboratory (sterile) lice to feed on
                  patient
                  Incubate lice
                  Isolate rickettsia from lice fecal matter
    Serology -   Complement - fixation
                  Immunofluorescent Antibody Test
                  Passive hemagglutination

CATCH SRATCH Fever (handwritten)

Treatment:
    Non-directed
    Chloramphenicol - rickettsiostatic

Epidemiology:
    Seen in World War I and II

NAME OF DISEASE: Q-Fever (Query-Fever)

Causative Organism: Coxiella burnettii

Characteristics of Organism:
        See Epidemic typhus

        Notable Features: Grows in vacuoles of infected cells
                                 Transmitted via fomites
                                 Two forms -   large
                                               small endospore-like
                                               structures

Portal of Entry:
        Inhalation from diseased animals
        Unpasteurized milk ingestion
        Eggs
        In animals-vector also is a tick

Clinical Symptoms:
        Incubations - two weeks
        An acute, febrile disease
        Dry, non-productive cough
        Fever - 103°-105°F
        Headache
        Muscle stiffness
        Liver enlarged tender lesions form containing:
                lymphocytes
                plasma cells
                giant cells
                central necrosis

Complications:
        Bronchopneumonia
        Endocarditis in situation of previously damaged heart
        valves - formation of vegetation - 2-20 years later

Diagnosis:
        Serology -   Aggulationation Test
                     Complement - Fixation

107

Treatment: Tetracycline and Lincomycin
              Fluoroquinolone

Epidemiology:
    First described in Queensland, Australia
    In 1940's limited to California
    Almost to east coast - 1990
    Transmitted to farmers during lambing
    Aerosolic blood - flu like symptoms
    Spring/Fall
    Untreated/inadequate   treatment-long   remissions   -
        cortisones will reactivate

108

CHLAMYDIAL DISEASES

Psittacosis
Trachoma
Inclusion Conjunctivitis
Non-gonococcal urethritis
Lymphogranuloma Venereum

More common in Women than Men

NAME OF DISEASE: **Psittacosis**
OTHER NAME(S):   **Parrot Fever**
                      Extension to all birds-ornithinosis

Causative Organism: <u>**Chlamydia**</u> <u>**psittaci**</u> *← Genus Species*
                      (Previous names of genus,
                      <u>**Rickettsiaformis Prowazekii**</u>**,**
                      <u>**Miyagawanella**</u>**,** <u>**Bedsonia**</u>**, Large virus,**
                      Basophilic viruses)

Characteristics of Organism:
    (small structure -
       infectious elementary
       body
    large structure -
       non-infectious initial
       body)

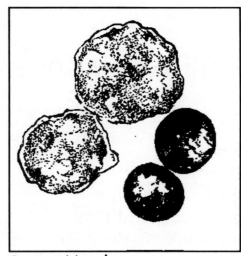

<u>**C. psattaci**</u>

    Group B -
       Chlamydia
       Diffuse inclusion body
       Lack of glycogen
       Does not stain with
         iodine
       Resistant to sulfa
         drugs
    Obligate intracellular parasite-lack ATP-generating
    mechanisms
    Spherical, gram-negative
    Non-motile
        Life cycle -   Outside host - Elementary body
                      200-300 nanometers
                      Absorbed/phagocytized by host cell
                      Enlarges into inclusion (initial)
                      body - 1000 nanometers
                      Grows/Divides
                      Reorganization into elementary body
                      Released to reinfect

Large virus size of viruses 20-250 outside of host cell

Portal of Entry:
      Respiratory: aerosolic bird feces
      Direct contact with droppings

Clinical Symptoms:
      In diseased birds:
            diarrhea
            emaciation
            mucopurulent discharge from nose
      In humans:
            Incubation 6-15 days
            Abrupt onset
            Headache/Fever - initially
            Backache
            Initially - non-productive cough
                changes to thick mucoid sputum
                (bronchopneumonia)
            Effects - liver, heart, spleen
            Faint macular rash - Horder's spots
            Hepatosplenomegaly
            Crepitant rales
            Tachypnea
            Alveolar exudate - initially-fibrin, enyhrocytes,
                neutrophils later - mononuclear lymphocytes
            Epithelial cells

Complications: Neurological
                  Encephalitis
                  Facial paralysis
                  Polyneuritis

Diagnosis:
      Cytology - Isolation of Chlamydia
              Stains: dark blue - Giemsa
                    red against blue - Gimenez
                        Machiavello
      Serology - Complement-fixation

111

Treatment:

    Tetracycline
    Penicillin for secondary bacterial infection
    Sulfadiazine will reduce severity

    Birds: Chlortetracycline in food

Epidemiology:
    Control - Isolate diseased birds
            Control of pet bird market
            Tighter regulation on importation of poultry - recent outbreaks with turkeys
    Female/male ration - 2/3
    Occupational risk

quarantined

Other -   Chlamydial pneumonia caused by <u>C. psatlaci</u>, TWAR (Taiwan, acute respiratory) renamed <u>C. pneumonae</u>
        Transmission - person to person
        Resembles mycoplasmal pneumonia
        Diagnosis - Fluorescent Antibody Test
        Treatment - Tetracycline

NAME OF DISEASE: Trachoma
OTHER NAME(S):   Granular conjunctivitis, keratoconjunctivitis

Causative Organism: <u>Chlamydia</u> <u>trichomatous</u>
                    (the TRIC agent)
                    TR - Trachoma
                    IC - Inclusion conjunctivitis

Characteristics of organism:
        Group A - chlamydia
                compact inclusion body
                presence of Glycogen
                sensitive to sulfa drugs
                stains with Iodine
                spherical/gram-negative
                non-motile
                reproductive cycle - see Psittacosis

Portal of Entry:
        Contract - direct
                indirect via fomites-towels, swimming pools
                vector - house fly

Clinical Symptoms:
        Incubation - 5 to 7 days
        Initially -
                I n f l a m m a t o r y
                    conjunctivitis
                Epithelial hyperplasia
                Hyperemia
                L y m p h o c y t i c
                    infiltration
                F o r m a t i o n   o f
                    lymphoid
                Follicles
        Progressive -
                Glandular crypts in conjunctiva
                Papillary hypertrophy

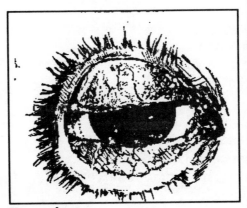

Traechoma

Short Incubation Period

113

Invasion of cornea by:
    blood vessels
    fibroblasts
Forms a pannus
Followed by necrosis and scarring
Usually upper eyelid involved

Complications:
    Secondary bacterial infections
    Blindness - 1st or 2nd (including Vitamin A deficiency)
    cause of preventable blindness
    15-20,000,000 cases of blindness out of 350-400,000,000 cases
    of trachoma/year

10% of the world

Diagnosis:
    Clinical picture
    Cytology - cells scraped from conjunctiva
                stain - Geimsa or iodine
                observe - inclusions
    Serology - eye secretions
                Fluorescent Antibody Test

Treatment:
    Topical tetracycline
    Topical sulfonamides
    Erythromycin ointment
    About 3 weeks

could correct with surgery

Epidemiology
    Highest incidence in Egypt and Sudan
    Highest incidence in United States
            Southwestern Indian reservations
            Appalachia
    Predisposition - poverty
                   malnutrition
                   poor hygiene

NOTES:

NAME OF DISEASE: Inclusion conjunctivitis
OTHER NAME(S): Inclusion blennorrhea (infants)
Swimming pool conjunctivitis (adults)
Paratrachoma

Causative Organism: Chlamydia trichomatous also referred to as
Chlamydia oculogenitalis

Characteristics of Organisms: See Trachoma

Portal of Entry:
Contact -   direct - coitus
contaminated hands
indirect - fomites
Passage through vaginal canal

Clinical symptoms:
Incubation - 5 to 12 days
Commonly effects lower lid (trachoma usually upper)
Copious macoprurulent discharge
In infants - 3-4 days after birth as opposed to gonorrhea in the 1-2 day range
Pannus/necrosis - non-existent
Adults - milder inflammation
Minimal mucopurulent discharge

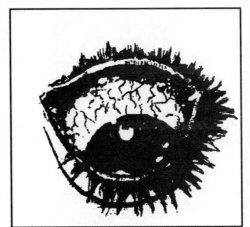

Conjunctivitis

Diagnosis:
Same as trachoma
Inclusions found in cells not pus

Treatment:
      Infants: Erythromycin drops
                 Tetracycline drops
      Adults: Antibiotic ointment

Epidemiology:
      Under chlorinated swimming pools containing genital discharges

NAME OF DISEASE: Non-gonococcal urethritis
OTHER NAME(S):   NGU, Non-specific urethritis, NSU

Causative Organism: Chlamydia trichomatous
                     also called C. oculogenitalis

Characteristics of Organism:
        See trachoma

Portal of Entry: Sexually transmitted

Clinical Symptoms:
        Male: non-copious, watery discharge
                  burning sensation on urination
                  urethral itching
                  48-96 hours after exposure
                  Untreated - Epididymitis
        Female: cervicitis
                  salpingitis
                  no or rare outward manifestation

Complications:
        Infertility
        Pelvic Inflammatory Disease in females

Diagnosis:
        Cultivation of organism is tissue culture (difficult)

Treatment: Tetracycline (does not respond to penicillin)

clear
sterility

some bleeding
scaring tissue

NAME OF DISEASE: Lymphogranuloma Vernrum
OTHER NAME(S): LGV, lymphogranuloma inguinale, tropical bubo, paradentitis, esthiomite, Duran-Nicholas-Favre Disease

Causative Organism: <u>Chlamydia</u> <u>trichomatous</u>
also called <u>C.</u> <u>Lymphogranulomatous</u>

Group B

Characteristic or Organism:
See Trachoma

Portal of Entry: Transmitted Sexually

Starts as small pimple

Clinical Symptoms:
Incubation - 7 to 12 days
Begins as small painless papule
Enlargement of lymph nodes balled buboes
Involvement of inguinal and femoral lymph nodes may produce "groove-sign" (nodes visibly separated via inguinale ligament)
Lymph nodes like granulomas
In center - neutrophils/necrosis

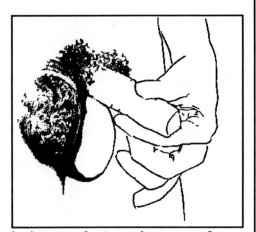

buboe of Lymphogranuloma venerum

Next zone of palisading epithelium
Macrophages and giant cells
Followed by lymphocytes, plasma vessel, fibrous tissue
Lymph node ulceration- seropurulent discharge - highly infectious
Lymph node involvement greater in male - leads to elephantiasis of genitals

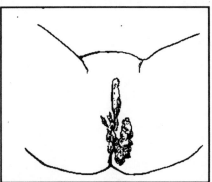

perianal lesions of lymphogranuloma venerum

In MALE - scrotum testes - large

condition of

In female - elephantiasis of vulva
anorectal fistulas
proctitis
tenesmus
diarrhea/bleeding
weight loss
Also -
   Fever
   bodyache
   conjunctivitis
   Central Nervous System Involvement

Complications:
   Meningo-encephalitis
   Sequelae -
      ulceration of penis, urethra, scrotum
      fistulas
      strictures of urethra
      ulcers of vulva
      smooth, pedunculated, perianal growths (lymphorroids)

untreated leads to

scar tissue will form

Diagnosis
   Serology -   Complement fixation
   Histology -   Increased WBC
                   Increased erythrocyte sedimentation
   Chemistry - Increased IgG
   Skin Test - Frei Test (no longer used in United States)

Treatment: Tetracycline
            Sulfonamide
            Cycloserine
            Damage Unrepairable

Epidemiology:
   More common - in tropical countries
                  in dark skin races
                  in males versus females (20/1)

Northeastern South America

British Guiana Dutch French

119

BACTERIAL INFECTIONS

VIA

RESPIRATORY ROUTE

Pneumococcal pneumonia (bacterial)
Staphylococcal pneumonia
Streptococcal pneumonia
Hemophilic pneumonia
Klebsiellan pneumonia
Primary Pneumonic Plague
Diphtheria
Pertussis
Listeriosis
Legionnaires Disease
Tuberculosis
Streptococcal Sore Throat
Scarlet Fever
Acute epiglottides
Nocardiosis
Bacterial Meningitis
Puerperal Fever
Impetigo Contagiosa
Erysipelas/cellulitis
Neonatal stretrococeal infection
Sequelae to streptococcal
Endocarditis
Subacute bacterial endocarditis
Rhinoscleroma
Sinusitis

NAME OF DISEASE: Pneumococcal pneumonia

Causative Organism: Steptoccus pneumiae
                              used to be called
                        Pneumococcus pneumonia

Characteristics of Organism:
    Group D streptoccus
    Gram - positive, lancet-shaped, pairs of cocci
    Dome-shaped colonies, smooth, mucoid, 1-2 mm
    Non-motile
    Non-spore forming
    Encapsulated -   his specific soluble substances (SSS)
                       83 antigenic types
                       polysaccharide antigens
    Ferments inulin-acid produced/no gas
    Catalase -   Negative
    Peroxide -   Negative
    Produces -   Hemolysins - alpha - hemolytic
                       Pneumolysis
                       Hyaluronidase
                       Leuocidins
    Delicate -   Does not survive in environment
    Culture -   prefers 5-10% CO_2

Portal of Entry:
    Respiratory route
            Droplet
            Contact - infective secretions

Predisposition:
    Trauma
    Viral infection
    Pulmonary disease
    Pulmonary edema
    Impaired phagocytosis
    Immunodeficiency

Clinical Symptoms:
    Incubation 1-3 days
    First two days inflammatory response
    Shaking chills/fever - 102° to 105° F
    Elevated pulse
    Thick scanty rust colored sputum
    Pleurisy
    Dyspnea - alveoli fill with fluid, RBC, WBC
    Malaise
    1-8 day neutrophilic inflammatory response
        Vascular enlargement
        Dilation of vessels
        Neutrophilic infiltration
        Followed by macrophages
    Extreme cases:
        Convulsions
        Cyanoses
        Delirium
    Lung sounds - dull, crackling sounds

Complications:
    Pleural effusion - fluid in chest
    Empyema - blood in thoracic cavity
    Septicemia
    Lung abscesses
    Meningitis - rare
    Endo - or pericarditis

Diagnosis:
    Cultural - organism from sputum
        on chocolate agar
        Blood Agar
        with increase carbon dioxide tension

Microscopic -   Gram - stain
                  Positive, cocci, in pairs

Serology -   Quelluning - Neufeld

X-Rays -   cloudiness, opacification - acute lobar
                  pneumonia - usually adults
                  children, elderly - bronchopneumonia

Special Tests -
    Fermentation of inulin
    Optochin Disc Test -   Disc contains
            ethyl-hydro cupreine HCl
            Swab agar plate with organism
            place disc on plate
            Lack of growth around disc
            a positive test
    Bile solubility Test
            Add sodium Deoxycholate to saline suspension of
            organisms.
            Contents clear-positive test

Treatment:
    Penicillin
    if allergic -   erythromycin
                           clindamycin
                           third generation cephalosporins

Epidemiology:
    In top 10 diseases that kill citizens in United States

    Type 3 -   most virulent
                      very thick capsule
                      evades phagocytosis
    Mortality -   Untreated 20%
                      Treated 1%
    Vaccine -   1977 - pneumovax
                      Effective against 14-23
                      antigenic types
                      for limited period

NAME OF DISEASE: Staphylococcal pneumonia

Causative Organism: <u>Staphylococcus</u> <u>aureus</u>

Characteristics of Organism:
    Gram-positive, cocci, in clusters
    Large round colonies on blood agar
    Alpha - hemolytic
    Non-spore forming
    non-motile
    Gelatin-positive
    Oxidase - positive
    Catalase - positive
    Non-encapsulated
    Colonies, round, raised yellow
    Cultured on mannitol salt-a selective media
    or EYA (egg-yolk agar) colonies appear
    Black with clear zone around them
    Stable - survives in pus
        pyogenic
        Resistant to disinfectants

Toxins:
Hemolysin   Fibrinolysin
Coagulase   Exfoliative toxins
Leucocidin   Enterotoxins
Hyaluronidase

Portal of Entry:
    Respiratory
    Other infections in body

Predisposition:
    Immunodeficient
    Viral infections
    Chronic lung disease
    Malignancy
    Broad - spectrum antibiotics

Diabetes / diseases of RES
Intranasal tubes
Excess I.V. fluid administration
Hematogenous

Clinical symptoms:
In adults -   High fever - 105-106°F
                          Cough with thick purulent yellow pus
                          Dyspnea/rales
                          Pleurisy
                          Consolidation and abscesses in lung
                          Hemorrhage/tissue destruction

In children -   Fever - lower (102°F)
                          Cyanosis/rapid breathing
                          Dry Cough
                          Pus-laden discharge - eyes and nose
                          Irritability
                          Expiratory grunting

Complications
    Empyema
    Shock/hypotension
    Coma

Diagnosis:
    X-ray - patchy infiltrates

    Microscopic - Gram - positive cocci in sputum

    Selective Media - Mannitol salt
    Coagulase Test
    Hematology - WBC elevated

Treatment:
    Antibiotic chosen after antibiotic sensitivity testing
    Initially -   methicillin, nafcillin
                              cephalosporin
                              allergic - I.V> vancomycin

125

Epidemiology:
    Control -   Handwashing
                 Carrier control - particularly
                      nurseries
                 Pus and such materials handled with care

126

NAME OF DISEASE: Streptococcal pneumonia

Causative Organism: Streptococcus pyogens
                        (Beta-hemolytic streptocci)

Characteristics of organism:
    Gram - positive, cocci, in chains
    Beta hemolytic
    Group A streptococci
    Facultative anaerobes
    Ferments - glucose and maltose
                        acid/no gas
    Non-motile
    Non-spore form
    Encapsulated - many antigenic types
    Produces -   Leucocidins
                        Hyaluronidase
                        Collagenase
                        Streptolysin
                        Streptodornase
                        Deoxyribonuclease
                        Streptokinase

Portal of Entry:
    Respiratory

Clinical Symptoms:
    Inflammatory response - rapid
    Infiltration edematous fluid
    Chills/Fever (102°-104°F)
    Cough/severe chest pain
    Sputum, purulent
    Dyspnea
    Malaise
    Hemorrhagic tissue destruction (necrosis)
    Fibrosis
    Consolidation of lung
    Mortality - untreated - 30%
                 treated - 5%

127

Complications:
    Endocarditis/pericarditis
    Meningitis - mortality - 50%
    Septicemia

Diagnosis:

Serology -	Quellung - neufeld
Microscopic -	Gram-positive cocci

Bacitracin Sensitivity Disc Test
            swab blood agar plate with organism
            place on disc
            lack of growth around disc - positive test

Treatment:
    Antibiotic Sensitivity Testing

NAME OF DISEASE: Hemophilic Pneumonia

Causative Organism: <u>Hemophilus</u> <u>influenza</u>
                        (Pfeiffer bacilli)

Characteristics of Organism:
   G r a m - n e g a t i v e ,
     coccobacillus
   1 x 0.3 micrometers
     (small)
   Aerobic
   Non-motile
   Non-spore forming
   Encapsulated -
     6 x antigenic types
     Type a through type f
   Growth requirements -
     X-V Factors
     X = hematin
     V = NAD

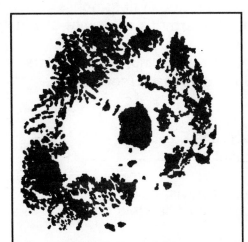

Epithelial cell with <u>Haemophilus influenza</u>

Portal of Entry:
   Respiratory route

Clinical Symptoms:
   Acute suppurative inflammatory response
     edema
     thick exudate
     broncho pneumonia
     minimal to no chills/fever

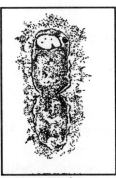

<u>Haemophilus influenza</u>, type B with motile capsule

Complications:

   Meningitis - Usually associated type b
              Small children
              Symptom - pain when child
              sits during diapering
              Fever
              Vomiting

Irritability/lethargy
Neurological defect in ⅓ that survive
Bacteria, neutrophils, fibrin
Compose exudate in leptomeninges
Bacteria reside in neutrophils
Bacteremia can lead to arthritis of weight bearing joints
Fever
erythema, swelling, heat at joints
pain or decreased movement

Diagnosis:
Culture -   Blood agar
Chocolate agar

Serology -   No hemolysis
Quelluning - newfeld

Hematology -   Leukocytosis - PMN's
leukopenia in severe infections

Treatment:
Ampicillin
Resistant strains - augmentin
Cefotaxime
Gentamicin

Epidemiology:
8-10,000 cases of meningitis in small children

Vaccine -   original only useful after the age of 2 years
Conjugate vaccine (newer) given as young as 2 months
Vaccine called Hib

NAME OF DISEASE: Klebsiellan Pneumonia
OTHER NAME(S):   Friedlander's pneumonia

Causative organism: <u>Klebsiella</u> <u>pneumonia</u>
                    (Friedlander's bacillus)

Characteristics of Organism:
    Gram-negative, bacillus
    Large, plump
    Non-motile
    Non-spore forming
    Encapsulated -
      14 antigenic types
    Exotoxin - damage lung

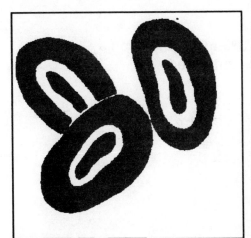

Encapsulated <u>Klebsiella</u>
<u>pneumoniae</u>

Portal of Entry:
    Respiratory route

Predisposition:
    Male alcoholics - over 40
           decreased phagocytic activity
           impaired cough reflex

    Malnutrition
    Chronically debilitate

Clinical Picture:
    Fever
    Pleurisy
    Cough - thick mucoid sputum
    Progresses -   shortness of breath
                    cyanosis
                    death ~2 to 3 days
    Mucous in alveoli - dominated by macrophages, Fibrin,
                    fluid compressed/necrotic abscesses
                    coalescent at cavitation

Treatment:
    Cephalosporins
    Gentamicin
    Tobramycin
    (response to therapy slow)

Epidemiology:
    Accounts for 1-3% of all pneumonia
    Mortality ~85% untreated

NAME OF DISEASE: Primary Plague Pneumonia

Causative Organism: Yersinia pestis
                        Used to be cased Pasteurella pestis

Characteristics of Organism:
     Gram-negative - coccobacillus
     Non-motile
     Non-spore forming
     Non-encapsulated
     Bipolar staining (safety - pin effect)
     Ferments -   galactose
                    levulose
                    maltose
                    mannose
                    acid produced/no gas

Portal of Entry:
     Respiratory route
     Break in skin (secondary plague pneumonia)
     Vector - flea
     Reservoir - rodents

Clinical Symptoms:
     Incubation 2 to 3 days
     High fever ~105°-106°F/chills
     Headache
     Tachycardia
     Tachypnea/dyspnea
     Productive cough -   first mucoid
                            then water, frothy

Diagnosis:
     Microscopic -   Specimens - sputum on blood agar
                       Gram stain
                       Wayson's stain (carbol fuchsin and methylene blue)

     Serology -   Fluorescent antibody

     Radiology -   Fulminating pneumonia

Treatment:
    Streptomycin
    or tetracycline, chloramphenicol,
    trimethoprim - sulfamethoxazole
    (must be started within 18 hours or onset of symptoms)

Epidemiology:
    Requires strict respiratory isolation
    Vaccine limited use - Haffkine
    Mortality -   100% untreated
                      18% treated

NAME OF DISEASE: Diphtheria
OTHER NAME(S):   Diphtheric pharyngitis

Causative Organism: <u>Corynebacterium</u> <u>diptheriae</u>
    (Klebs - Loeffler/ bacillus)

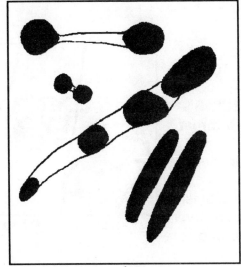

Characteristics of Organism:
    Gram - positive - 0.51-1 to
        5 micrometers
    Bacillus in palisades
        arrangement but
    also pleomorphic -
        clubs and dumb-bells
        granules - beaded
            appearance
    Facultative anaerobe
    Ferments glucose -
          Acid/no gas
    Non-motile -
        gelatin negative
    Non-spore forming
    Non-encapsulated
    Metachromatic granules - metaphosphate
        complexes - also called volutin
        granules - diagnostically important
    Catalase - positive
    Urease - negative
    Cultural media -   Loeffler's
            Cystine - Tellurate
            Pai's
    Exotoxin - 2 parts
        One prevents protein synthesis
           cells die
        Second effects heart and nervous system

    Produced only after bacteriophage infection
        called a lysogenic-conversion
        bacteriophage is beta-corynephage

Corynebacterium diptheriae

Portal of Entry:
    Respiratory Route
    Ingestion -
      contaminate food
      unpasteurized milk
    Host-human

Clinical Symptoms:
    Incubation - 1 to 10 days
      (7 average)
    Low fever 101°-102°F
    Unremarkable sore throat
    Progresses
    Lymadenopathy in neck -
      bull-neck
    Thick, patchy, grayish-
    green membrane over
    mucous membrane of
    throat

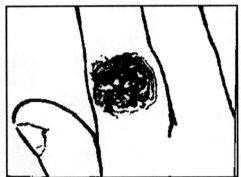
cutaneous diptheric ulcer

    Pseudomembrane composed of blood
      tissue exudates
      lymph
      fibrin
      dead cells
    Solidifies and can remain in place up to 3 weeks
    Sloughed off - if removed, bleeding occurs

Course of Disease:
    Bacteria grow on mucous membrane near tonsils. Toxins
    destroy cells, creating
    More favorable conditions for bacteria
    More toxin, more cells killed etc.

Complications:
    Toxemia
    Heart - myocarditis
        fatty degeneration
        murmurs
        arrhythmias
        failure

Central Nervous System
        Motor nerves more common then sensory nerves
        Loss of pupillary accommodation
        Paralysis of soft palate
        Alteration in voice
        Swallowing difficulties
        Paralysis
        Kidney - Nephritis
        Pneumonia

Diagnosis:
    2 steps
      1. Isolate organism
          Identify with Loeffler/s stain
          (alkaline methene blue)
      2. Determine if organism virulent
          (toxin producing)

Virulence determination
    In vivo -   0.I ml. into shave skin of mice
                One with antitoxins, the other not
                2 to 3 days - necrosis at injection
                site of unprotected
    In vitro -   agar - gel precipitin
                Elek's diffusion

Treatment:
    Even before confirmation
    Two steps
      1. Specific antitoxin
      2. Antibiotics - penicillin, erythromycin

Epidemiology:
    Skin sensitivity test - Schick
      0.I ml. of dilute diphtherial toxin
      (subcutaneous)

    Will redden and desquamation
    Areas turn brown
    Indicates susceptibility

Cutaneous form of Diphtheria
    Usually on limb or appendage
    Ulcer with raised, firm border
    base covered with membrane
    Necrotic
    Diphtheroids do not reach circulatory system

Other diptheroids
    C. pseudodiptheriticum -   normal flora of nose
        problem when artificial heart valves inplanted

    C. ulcerans, C pseudotuberculosis if
        converted can cause diphtheria
    Diphtheroid JK - high mortality rate
      associated with heart valves, IV catheters
    C. haemolyticum and C. ulcerans may
      cause pharyngitis like Group A streptocci

    on Tellurite media, three varieties of
    C. diphtheriae grow
        var. mitis -   smooth, convex, glossy colonies
        var. gravis -   semi-rough, flat, gray, large colonies
        var. intermedius - small, smooth, fried-egg appearance,
                       black colonies

Prevention -   Vaccine, part of DPT
           Booster not given to adults
           due to hypersensitivity
           Do Moloney test first -
              intradermal injection of diluted toxin or heated
              exotoxin

           Strict isolation of patient
              Organisms lives long time in
                saliva/mucous-even dry
              Disinfection important
              fibrinous membrane coughed
              out is contagious - on objects
              dries and becomes aerosolic

NAME OF DISEASE: Pertussis
OTHER NAME(S):   Whooping Cough

Causative Organism: <u>Bordetella</u> <u>pertussis</u>
                    (<u>Hemophilus</u> <u>pertussis</u>, Bordet-Gengou
                    bacillus)

Characteristics of Organism:
    Gram-negative, small bacillus
    Obligate pathogen
    Strict aerobe
    Hemolytic
    Non-motile
    Non-spore forming
    Encapsulated
    Media - Bordet -Gengou medium
        potato, blood, glycerol,
        peptone and penicillin
        (contaminates)
        Slow growth - 6 to 7 days
        37°C
        small, mercury drop-like colonies

    Toxins -   Exotoxin - heat labile
                    tracheal cytotoxin
                    effects ciliated cells

                Endotoxin - heat stable
                Lymphocytosis producing factor =
                histamine sensitizing factor

Portal of Entry:
    Respiratory Route

Course of Disease:
    Organism enters respiratory system
    Attaches to ciliated epithelium
    Simulate production of profuse, tenacious mucous

Local necrosis
Loss of ciliary ladder

Clinical Symptoms:
Incubation - 1 to 21 days (average 7)
3 stages
    1. Catarrhal stage -   Resembles flu
        bronchitis, cough, low or no fever,
        sneezing/coughing/lacrimation

    2. Paroxysmal
            Spasmodic coughing
            Rapid inspiration after coughing bout
            Creates whoop
            Vomiting due to swallowing mucous
            Hypoxia
            Clear, stringy mucous from nose
            10-15 attacks a day
            Exhaustion
    3. Convalescent stage -   less severe episodes
                               coughing
                               Recovery up to a year

Complications:
Pneumonia (secondary bacterial infection)
Convulsions
Hemorrhages
Atelectasis (collapsed lung)
Interstitial emphysema

Diagnosis:
Collection of Specimens
    Bordet-Gengou Cough Plate
    Nasopharyngeal swab

Serology -   Agglutination Test
                  Fluorescent Antibody Test

Treatment:
    Young - erythromycin (renders non-infectious)
    ampicillin
    trimethoprim - sulfamethoxazole

Epidemiology
    Vaccine -   Part of DPT
                 2, 4, 6 months, also 18 months
                 4 and 6 years - not beyond-causes
                 severe fever
                 Merthiolate - killed organism

    Related disease:
    Parapetusis
    Caused by <u>Bordetella</u> <u>parapertussis</u>

NAME OF DISEASE: Listeriosis
OTHER NAME(S):   Listeria meningitis

Causative Organism:
   Listeria monocytogenes

Characteristics of Organism:
   Gram - positive, coccobacillus in palisades
   young culture motile-through peritriculous
   flagella (1-4)
   Beta Hemolytic
   Non-spore forming
   Resistant to cold (grown in refrigerator) heat, ph, bile
   Catalase positive
   Forms black colonies on tellurite media
   (related to corynebacterium)
   Broad distribution in environment

Portal of Entry:
   Respiratory route
   Unpasteurized milk
   Direct contact

Predisposition:
   Very young
   Immunosuppressed
   Pregnant women
   Cancer patients

Clinical Symptoms:
   Adults -   Meningitis
                   Monocytosis
                   Septicemia
                   Shock with intravascular coagulation
                            endocarditis
   Organism grows in macrophages

   Neonates -   crosses placenta
                   most severe during third trimester
                   Neonatal sepsis -

Granulomatous infantiseptica
Meningitis
Irritability, convulsions, lethargy coma
Spontaneous abortion
Mortality as high as 50%

Other symptoms:
    Respiratory distress
    Hepatosplenomegaly
    Papular cutaneous lesions
    Mucosal lesions
    Leukopenia
    Thrombocytopenia

Diagnosis:
    Cultural -   In refrigerator - 4oC (incubate)
                      Blood agar
                      Motility Test (tumbling on wet mount)
                      Catalase test

    Serology -   Agglutination
                      Cervical swab - Fluorescent antibody

Treatment:
    Penicillin
    Ampicillin
    with gentamicin
    or tetracycline
        erthyromycin
        chloramphenicol

143

NAME OF DISEASE: Legionnaires Disease
OTHER NAME(S):   Legionellosis, Pontiac Fever

Causative Organism:
    Gram-negative, small pleomorphic bacillus
    Slow - growing
    Resistant to chlorine and heat
    special medias
        Charcoal agar extract-selective
        Hemoglobin/cystine agar
        Grow at 35°C, 2.5% CO_2
    Stains - gimenez silver impregnation

Portal of Entry:
    Respiratory

Clinical Symptoms:
    Incubation - 2 to 10 days
        Diarrhea
        Headache/muscle aches
        Dry cough
        Increased temperature
        Prostration
        Pulmonary consolidation
        Stridor
        Liver/kidney affected
        Lasts 1 - 16 days

Complications:
    Confusion / memory loss
    Impaired kidney function
    Cardiac damage

Diagnosis:
    Radiological -   Unilateral, diffuse bronchopneumonia
                    No cavitation

    Histology -   Formalin - fixed, paraffin - embedded
                    tissue - direct fluorescent antibody

Serology -   DNA probe
                 ELISA
                 Microagglutination

Treatment:
    Erythromycin with rifampin

Epidemiology:
    1000$^+$ reported per year
    Source -   stagnant water, showers, air conditioning and
                contaminated soil

NAME OF DISEASE: Tuberculosis
Causative Organism: <u>Mycobacterium</u> <u>tuberculosis</u>
         (Koch's bacillus)

Characteristics of Organism:
    Gram- positive, but takes
        stain poorly
    Acid - Fast (diagnostically
        important)
    0.5 by 3 micrometers
    Long slender, straight or
        curved bacilli
    Granular and vacuoles
    Non-encapsulated
    Non-spore forming
    Non-motile
    Strict aerobes
    Resistant to drying and

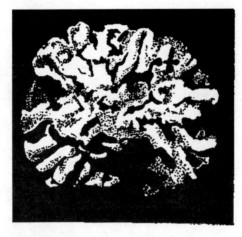

Mycobacteium colony

    Sunlight, many
        disinfectants
    Pigmented
    Sinuous cords -   2 components
            complex wax (lipid) portion
            cord factor
            leucotoxic portion-prevents
            phagocytosis
            heat sensitive
    Stains -   Ziehl - Neelson
            Kinyoun
    Cultural -   Many specialized medias
            Lowenstein - Jenson
            Middlebrook oleic acid
            Cohn's
            Petragnani
            Targhish blood
            Dubos
            Slow growing
            Generation time - 20 hours

Incubation
    8-13 weeks at
    37° and 3-10% carbon dioxide
Colonies - yellow to cream
    colored, wrinkled rough granular

Portal of Entry:
    Respiratory route
        Direct-Infective   dose
            low
        Very infectious
        Indirect-fomites
        I n g e s t i o n   -
            unpasteurized milk

Predisposition:
    Malnutrition
    Poor sanitation/ventilation
    Age - extremes
    Chronic   alcoholism   -
        reduced phagocytosis
    Metabolic   disease   -
        e.g. diabetes
    Prolonged stress

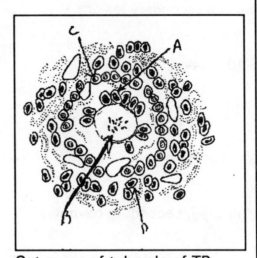

Cut away of tubercle of TB
A-multinucleated giant cells
B-caseous necrosis
C-epitheliod cells
D-granuloma cells

Course of Disease:
    Organism to lung
    Exudative stage -   Inflammation
    Productive stage -   Immune response
                3-4 weeks to establish
                formation of tubercle
                (granuloma)
                Overall consists of
                fibroblasts, neutrophils,
                lymphocytes and multinucleated giant cells
                (Langhan's cells)
                Cell-mediated response
    Caseation -   center becomes cheesy
                tissue coagulation

147

Heal -   calcium deposits/scaring
                  radiology - Ghon complex
Resolution -   Disappearance of infiltrating macrophage
Other possibilities
    Disseminated via blood to other parts of the body or latent
    (dormant) produces secondary lesions

Clinical Symptoms:
    Incubation - 2 to 10 weeks
    Chronic cough
    Thick, rust-colored sputum
    Hemoptysis
    Pleurisy
    High fever - peaks in afternoon
    Weight loss

Secondary (acute adult-type, secondary cavitary)
    Cough
    Low grade fever
    General malaise
    Anorexia
    Night sweats
    Histologically - tubercle enlarges
    Central area is necrotic
    Spreads to bronchial tube
    Contents spill into airway -
     migration to larynx
    Tubercle may fill with air
    Radiology -lesions round,
      cavity
        "coin lesion"
    Pleural fibrosis adhesions

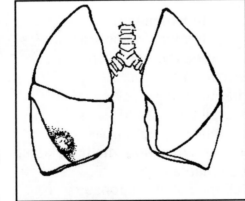

Tubercle of TB

Complications:
    T.B. of spine - Pott's
       Disease
            leads to kyphosis,
              lordosis
    T.B. of peritoneum
    T.B. meningitis - retardation, blindness, deafness

T.B. of kidney - necrosis, scarring, hematuria
Miliary tuberculosis (chronic disseminated
    tuberculosis, consumption)
    Hematogenic dispersal
    Small grains beneath skin - like
    millet seeds - hence name
        loss of weight
        cough
        loss of vigor

Diagnosis:
    Specimens- Catherized urine
        CSF
        Pleural Fluids
        Tissue biopsy
        Sputum
            Collection elderly - tracheal suction
                nebulization
            (Hypertonic saline)
            Mucous exposed to NaOH
                (kill bacteria)
            N-acetylcystein - dissolves
                mucin
            Stain - acid fast
                auramine, O
                rhodamine
    Serology - Fluorescent antibody
            Chromatography - fatty acids
            DNA probes

Treatment:
    Tripartite drugs regimen

Choices
    INH (isoniazid)   Pyrazinamide
    rifampin   Thiacetazone
    PAS   Caporemycin
    Ethambutol   Kanamycin
    Streptomycin   Ethionamide
    Thiorectazone

Epidemiology:
　　Skin sensitivity tests -
　　　　allergen is PPD - purified protein derivative
　　　　used to be OT - Old tuberculin
　　Different formats of presentation
　　　　Mantoux - intradermal
　　　　Heaf - multiple puncture
　　　　Tine - multiple puncture
　　　　Vollmer - gauze patch, superficial
　　　　von Pirquet - scarification
　　48 hours later - induration - hard, small lesions

Incidence - world wide　　　　20-25 million cases
　　　　　　　　　　　　　　　　4-5 million new cases per year
　　　　　　　　　　　　　　　　300,000 + deaths per year

Terminology of Disease states -
　　Active -　organisms in specimens
　　　　　　　x-rays - positive
　　　　　　　subgroups - active, unimproved
　　　　　　　　　　　　　active, improved

　　Inactive
　　　　Inactive, non-cavitary - negative bacterio -
　　　　　　　logical/radiological results - 6 months
　　　　Inactive, cavitary - cavity increases
　　　　　　　bacterial results - negative 18 months
　　　　Quiescent - non-cavitary and cavitary

Activity Undetermined

Classification of Mycobacterium
　　Runyon Groups based on - color, growth rate

Group I -　　Photochromogens - yellow/slow growth
Group II -　　Scotochromogens - yellow orange/slow growth
Group III -　Nonchromogens - no pigment/slow growth
Group IV -　Rapid growers - no pigment

Other mycobacterial diseases

<u>M</u>. <u>aviuvm</u> -	Seen in AIDS patients
	very severe
	doesn't respond well to drug regimen
	Lesions on blood vessels
	Hemorrhage
	Blood in sputum
<u>M</u>. <u>bovis</u> -	Respiratory tuberculosis
	miliary tuberculosis
	peritoneal tuberculosis
<u>M</u>. <u>fortuitum</u> -	Ocular/skin lesions
<u>M</u>. <u>kansasii</u> -	Non-tubericuliod lesions of lung
<u>M</u>. <u>marinium</u> -	"Swimming pool granuloma"
	cutaneous lesions
	Satellites along lymphatics
	Nodules ulcerate
	Early - neutrophils
	Histiocyles, lymphocytes
	late - tuberculoid granulomas
<u>M</u>. <u>ulcerans</u> -	Suppurative granulomas of skin
<u>M</u>. <u>scrofulameum</u> -	Scrofula in children
	enlarge lymph nodes, ulcerate
	and drain

<u>Mycobacterium</u> <u>ulcerans</u> -

          Buruli ulcer
          Route-minor penetrating wounds on limbs at joints
          Cytotoxin diffuses symmetrically
          Lesions - firm, painless
          Become papular - then ulcer
          scalloped, deep
          Healing - long time
          Destruction of collagen

NAME OF DISEASE: Streptococcal sore throat
OTHER NAME(S):   "Strep", strep throat, streptococcal
pharyngitis

Causative Organism: **Streptococcus** **pyogens**

Characteristics of Organisms:
    Gram-positive cocci in chains
    Non-motile
    Non-spore forming
    Moderately resistant to environmental factors
    Sensitive to disinfectants
    Fermentative - non-oxygen environment
    Ferment glucose/maltose--acid /no gas
    Catalase negative

Two classification schemes
  1. Based on Hemolysis - Sherman's
      Alpha-hemolytic -partial breakdown
      Beta - hemolytic - complete breakdown
      Gamma - hemolytic - no hemolysis

  2. Based on Antigenicity
    Lancefield's Two Antigens
      C - carbohydrate antigen
      divides in 18 groups
      Identified A-R
      M-protein (Griffith)
      Types using numerical subscripts

Toxins - Virulence Factors
  Carbohydrate - necrosis of myocardium
               prevents lysis
    LTA (lysoteichoic acid) attaches bacteria to cells

    M-protein - antiphagocytic adherence

Streptolysin O and S - Breakdown RBC's
　　intravascular hemolysis
　　induces arthritis
　　renal tuberlar necrosis

Erythrogenic toxin - causes rash
　　due to lysogenic conversion
Streptokinase - dissolve clots
Streptodornase - damages DNA
Hyaluronidase - spreading factor
Leucocidin - destroys WBC

Portal of Entry:
Respiratory
　　Direct - human/pets
　　　fomites - food, milk, water

Clinical Symptoms:
　　Short Incubation - 1 to 5 days
　　Fever - 101°-104°F
　　Sore Throat
　　Beefy red pharynx
　　Swollen lymph nodes
　　Tonsil swell, white, pus-filled lesions
　　Little nasal discharge /no cough

Complications:
　　Otitis media
　　Sequelae - if not treated properly
　　　　rheumatic fever
　　　　glomerulonephritis
　　　　erythema nodosum

Diagnosis:
　　Cultural -　　　Throat culture on blood agar
　　　　　　　　　beta hemolysis
　　Hematology -　Elevated WBC
　　Serology -　　Bacitracin sensitivity test
　　Kit -　　　　Rapid Streptococcal Antigen
　　　　　　　　　Detection kit

Treatment:
Penicillin
Erythromycin

Epidemiology:
Other Diseases
1. Erysipelas - (St. Anthony's Fire)
Reddened, swollen, lesions
spread but sharply defined
Face/scalps
Rupture - yellowish fluid
Stinging/itching
Fever
Lymadnopathy - spread to lymphatics

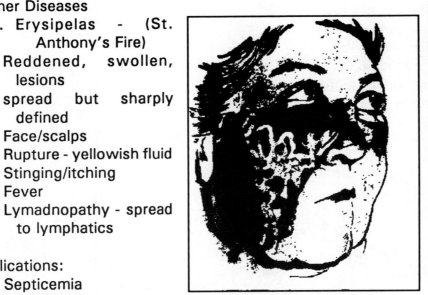

Streptococcal erysipelas

Complications:
Septicemia
Endocarditis
Arthritis
Pneumonia
Abscesses

NAME OF DISEASE: Scarlet Fever
OTHER NAME(S):   Scarlatina

Causative Organism: Streptococcus pyogenes
                          (Streptococcus scarlatina)

Characteristics of Organism:
    See Streptococcal sore throat

Portal of Entry:
    Respiratory Route

Clinical Symptoms:
    Incubation - 1 to 10 days
    Goose pimple rash - fades with pressure
        first on back/chest spreads within 36 hours
        During convalescence - desquamation

        Adenopathy
        Via blood to joints, bones, endocardium
        Changes in tongue
            Furry coating
            into "strawberry" tongue
            into "raspberry" tongue
            (red, enlarged, loss of outer membranes)
        High fever - 101°-104°F

Complications:
    Rheumatic fever
    Glomerulonephritis
    Erythema nodosum
    Deafness

Diagnosis:
    See streptococcal sore throat

Treatment:
    Penicillin
    Erythromycin

Epidemiology:
    Skin Sensitivity Test - Dick Test
        intradermal introduction of toxin

    Diagnostic Skin Test - Schick Test
        intradermal injection of antitoxin into rash
        blanches - positive

    Most common - temperate regions
        fall, winter, spring
        causians
        children under 10

NAME OF DISEASE: Acute Epiglotitidis
OTHER NAME(S):   Obstructive laryngotracheal obstruction

Causative Organism:
    See Hemophiliac pneumonia

Portal of Entry:
    Respiratory

Clinical Symptoms:
    Severe, red, edematous throat
    Obstructs respiration
    Low grade fever
    Mostly children from ½ - 2½ years old

Complications:
    Meningitis

Treatment:
    Tracheostomy if needed
    Penicillin
    Tetracycline
    Chloramphenicol

157

NAME OF DISEASE: Nocardiosis

Causative Organism: <u>Nocardia</u> <u>asteroides</u>

Characteristics of Organism:
    gram - positive, branching
        filaments
    aerobic
    weakly acid fast
    stains silver impregnation
        techniques
    cultured on Sabourauds -
        wrinkled colony

Portal of Entry:
    Respiratory

Clinical Symptoms:
    Bronchopneumonia -
        night sweats
        fever
        weight loss
        cough
        lesions - diffuse
            necrotic centers

Complications:
    Spreads to brain

Treatment:
    Sulfadiazine + sulfisoxazole or
    Sulfonamide + Trimethoprin
    with drugs less than 50% mortality
    Treatment 6 weeks to 1 year

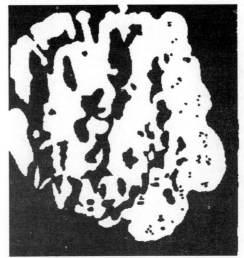

<u>Nocardia</u> <u>asteroides</u> colony at
room temperature on
Sabouraud's

NAME OF DISEASE: Bacterial Meningitis
OTHER NAME(S):   Cerebrospinal Fever, epidemic
                        cerebrospinal meningitis

Causative Organism: <u>Neisseria</u> <u>meningitides</u>

Characteristics of Organism:
    Gram-negative - diplococci
        kidney-bean shaped forming a donut appearance
    Non-motile/non-spore forming
    Sensitive to drying, cold, acidity, light
    aerobic/microaerophilic
    Catalase positive
    Oxidase - positive
    Ferment - glucose
            maltose
           acid /no gas
    Protease - positive
              cleaves IgA on mucous membrane
              virulence factor
    Pili present -   attachment to epithelium
                   reduce phagocytosis
                   virulence factor
    Encajgvaleted -   antigenic types (13)
                   Major types - A,B,C,D
                   other types - X,Y,Z,29EW,135
    Medias -   Chocolate Agar - small, glistening,
                       translucent colonies
             Thayer - Martin
             Martin - Lewis

Portal of Entry:
    Respiratory Route

Clinical Symptoms:
    Nasopharyngitis -   Asymptomatic
    Meningitis -   Fever - high
                    Headache
                    Stiffness in back of neck
                    Rigidity of neck

Rash -begins bright red
        turns purple to black
Delirium/confusion
coma
Children - early chills, irritability, vomiting

Septicemia -   Spiking fever/chills
        Headache
        Sore throat
        cough
        myalgia/arthralgia
        Tachypnea - mild
        Maculapaploar rash

Meningococcemia -   via endotoxin
        Fever
        Hypotension
        Tachycardia
        Leucocytosis or leucopenia
        Clogging of blood vessel
        Thrombocytopenia
        Intravascular coagulation
        Adrenal failure
        Joint pain
        Skin hemorrhages
        Splenomegaly
        Respiratory or cardiac failure

Complications:
  Residual CNS effects -   Convulsions
        Deafness
        Blindness
        Paralysis
        Mental deterioration
        (Institutionalization)

Diagnosis:
    Specimens -   blood, CSF, nasophorygeal swab
    Oxidase Test -   colony treated with
                         tetraethyl-p-phenylenediamine
                         HCl - color change
                         Pink to magenta or dark red to black
    Microscopic -   Diplococci in leucocyles

    Serology - Fluorescent antibody test
                 Counter immunoelectrophoresis
                 Rapid latex agglutination tests

Treatment:
    Begin before confirmation
        Penicillin
        Chloramphenicol
        Tetracycline
        Erythromycin
        Ceftroxime
        Cloxycycline
        For meningococcemia - sulfadiazine

Epidemiology:
    Mortality -Untreated 85%, treated 17%
    2-3,000 cases per year
    Predisposition - overcrowding
                        temperature/humidity
                        fatigue
                        lack of immunity
    Vaccine -   type A and C
                       against cell wall polysaccharide
                       antigen
                       Limited effectiveness

Waterhouse - Friderichsen Syndrome
    Immunological response - possibly due to
       different antigenic types
    Hemmorrahgic lesions in adremals

Hormonal imbalances
Clotting of blood
Purpura
Circulatory collapse

Other types Meningitis
Hemophilic -   48% of cases, up to 20,000
                per year, Mortality less than 30% - treated
Leading cause of mental institutionalization
possible permanent CNS damage

Pneumococcal -   13% of cases
                  Mortality - 21-40%
Spirochetal -   2 forms - Leptospiral - benign
                 treponemal - malignant
                 Mucosal route
Anaerobic bacterial -   Bacteroides, anaerobic
                         streptococcus
                         wounds to head
Neonatal -   Gram negative enterics,
              Listeria, staphylococcus, hemolytic
              streptococci
Viral -   Aseptic/benign
Fungal - Progressive and fatal

NAME OF DISEASE: Puerperal Fever
OTHER NAME(S):   Child-bed fever, post-partum fever

Causative Organism: <u>Streptococcus pyogenes</u>

Characteristics of Organism:
   See Streptococcal sore throat

Portal of Entry:
   Vaginal - indirect
     fomites -   contaminated hands
                contaminated instruments

Clinical Symptoms:
   Fever
   Malaise
   Uterine tenderness

Complications:
   Septicemia
   Toxic shock syndrome

Diagnosis:
   Specimens vaginal swab/blood

Treatment:
   Penicillin

NAME OF DISEASE: Impetigo contagiosa
OTHER NAME(S): Streptococcal pyoderma

Causative Organism: <u>Streptococcus</u> <u>pyogenes</u>
another cause <u>Staphylococcus</u> <u>aureus</u>

Characteristics of Organism:
See streptococcal sore throat

Portal of Entry:
Direct Contact

Clinical Symptoms:
Macules develop into vesicles
Become pustular
Scab
Secondary erythema
Itching (scratching spreads disease)
Dense depigmented regions

Complication:
Glomerulonephritis

Diagnosis:
See streptococcal sore throat

Treatment:
Tetracycline
Penicillin
Erythromycin
Clindamycin
(orally or topically)

NAME OF DISEASE: Erysipelas/cellulitis
OTHER NAME(S): St. Anthony's Fire

Causative Organism: <u>Streptococcus</u> <u>pyogenes</u>

Characteristics of Organism:
    See Streptococcal sore throat

Portal of Entry:
    Wound/break in skin

Clinical Symptoms:
    Red, swollen raised lesions
    (face/scalp)
    Surround small vesicles, easily ruptured,
    containing thin yellowish fluid
    Stinging, itching
    Fever
    Headache
    Cervical lymadenopathy

    Cellulitis
    Rapid spread
    Swelling
    Spreads to subcutaneous tissue
    Lymphangitis - notable by red streaking
    Can be fatal

Diagnosis:
    See Streptococcal sore throat

Treatment:
    Penicillin

NAME OF DISEASE: Neonatal stretrococeal infection

Causative Organism: <u>Streptococcus</u> <u>agalacticace</u>

Characteristics of Organism:
    See Streptococcal sore throat
    5 antigenic types
    Inhabits genitals and gastrointestinal tracts

Portal of Entry:
    Direct contact

Clinical Symptoms:
    Neonatal septicemia
        Early - onset- pneumonia
                    bacteremia
                    meningitis
                    affects premature babies

        Late - onset- bacteremia
                    meningitis
                    bone/joint involvement
                    mortality less than 15%
                    seizure

Diagnosis:
    Specimens - blood, CSF, skin
    Isolate Group B streptococci

Treatment:
    Penicillin
    Ampicillin

NOTES:

NAME OF DISEASE: Sequelae to Streptococcal Infections
                    Rheumatic Fever
                    Glomerulonephritis - acute (AGN)
                    Erythema nodosum

Portal of Entry:
    Mechanism hypersensitivity reaction

Clinical Symptoms:
    Rheumatic Fever - 14-28 days after infection
        Chronic disease of heart -mitral/aortic stenosis or
        insufficiency
    Evidenced by murmurs
    Mostly in children - 3 to 15
    Damage to heart valves - via formation of Aschoff bodies
    Other symptoms-   polyarthritis
                       sore throat
                       subcutaneous lesions
                       fever
                       less than 10% develop
                       Sydenham's chorea or
                       St. Vitus Dance -
                       involuntary flailing
                       of limbs - need restraint

Acute Glomerulonephritis
    (Acute hemorrhaging or Bright's Disease)
        Hematuria
        Proteinuria
        Edema
                Hypertension
                Fever
Erythema nodosum
        Tender subcutaneous lesions
        Fever

Treatment:
    Anti - inflammatory
    Antibiotics as needed, such as before surgery

167

NAME OF DISEASE: Endocarditis
OTHER NAME(S): Acute Endocarditis

Causative Organism: Group D streptococci (enterococci)
Streptococcus durans
Streptococcus faecalis
Streptococcus faecium

Characteristics of Organism:
6.5% NaCl in media
otherwise - see streptococcal sore throat

Portal of Entry:
Breaks in skin

Predisposition:
Elderly
Wounds
Surgery
Urinary Tract
Infection

Clinical Symptoms:
Weakness/fatigue
Fever
Night sweats
Arthralgia
Splenomegaly

Diagnosis:
Anemia
Increase immunoglobulins
Culture - see subacute bacterial endocarditis

Treatment:
Penicillin or
Ampicillin with aminoglycoside

NAME OF DISEASE: Subacute bacterial endocarditis

Causative Organism: <u>Streptococcus</u> <u>viridans</u>

Characteristics of Organism:
Alpha - hemolytic
Otherwise - See Streptococcal sore throat

Portal of Entry:
Other bacterial infections foci
Bacteria lodge in damaged tissue of heart

Clinical Symptoms:
Fever
Amena
Weakness
Emboli
Formation of vegetation on valves
Regurgitating heart murmur
Congestive heart failure

Diagnosis
Differentiate - cAMP factor, Bacitracin sensitivity,
Esculin hydrolysis, SXT sensitivity growth in broth, at 45°C,
Meida 6.5% salt. Rapid direct test kits.

Treatment:
Long term penicillin

NAME OF DISEASE: Rhinoscleroma

Causative Organism: <u>Klebsiella rhinoscleromitis</u>

Characteristics of Organism:
  Gram-negative
  Non-motile
  Non-spore forming
  Encapsulated

Portal of Entry
  Respiratory route

Clinical Symptoms:
  Starts as cold
  Nasal mucosa becomes reddish, waxy
  Granulomatous infiltration of mucosa
  Hard nodular intranasal masses
  Changes to aloe and tip of nose
    (Mebra nose)
  Airway obstruction
  Anosmia
  Speech difficulties
  Destruction of bone
  Anesthesia of soft palate
  Damaged tissue replaced by scar tissue

Treatment:
  Streptomycin
  Tetracycline
  Chloramphenicol
  Surgery - practical/cosmetic

NAME OF DISEASE: Sinusitis

Causative Organism: <u>S</u>. <u>pneumonia</u>, <u>H</u>. <u>influenza</u>
                                    <u>S</u>. <u>aureus</u>, <u>S</u>. <u>pyogenes</u>

Clinical Symptoms:
    Acute -   Swelling impedes drainage
                      Results pressure/pain
                      Mucous builds up, a media for
                          bacterial growth
                      Phagocytes chemotactically attracted
                          to region

    Chronic -   Permanent damage
                      Pendulous growths or polyps

Treatment:
    Moist heat
    Vasocontrictors like ephedrine
    Humidification
    Pain - killers - codeine
    Penicillin - if other techniques fail

Epidemiology:
    Frequently seen in underwater divers -
    Frequently forcing water up nose - possible source of infection

Bacterial Disease

of

Oral Cavity

Actinomycosis
Necrotizing Ulcerative Gingivitis

NAME OF DISEASE: Actinomycosis
OTHER NAME(S):   Lumpy jaw, Ludwig's Angina

Causative Organism: <u>Actinomyces</u> <u>israelis</u>
    <u>Actinomyces</u> <u>bovis</u>
    <u>Actinomyces</u> <u>nesejslundii</u>
    <u>Actinomyces</u> <u>viscosus</u>
    <u>Archnia</u> <u>proprionica</u>
    <u>Bifidobacterium</u> <u>adolecentis</u>

Characteristics of Organism:
    Gram-positive - filamentous
    Part of normal flora
    Facultative anaerobe

Portal of Entry:
    Wounds

Clinical Symptoms:
    Cervico - facial-
        red swelling
        hard lumps
        draining sinuses
        sulfur granules-
        yellow-gray
        masses - colonies

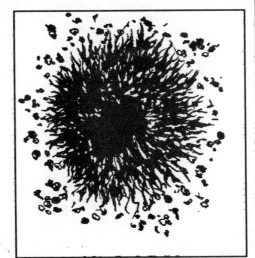

Sulfur granules
<u>Actinomyces</u>

    Respiratory - Fever
        atelectasis
        productive cough
        hemoptysis
        empyema
        draining sinuses
    Also effects brains, bone, female reproductive tract

Diagnosis:
    Presence of sulfur granules in biopsy tissue

Treatment:
    Penicillin over 6 weeks
    Tetracycline 6-12 months
    Surgical drainage

NAME OF DISEASE: Necrotizing Ulcerative Gingivitis
OTHER NAME(S):　　NUG, Fusospirochetal disease
　　　　　　　　　　trench mouth, Vincent's angina (pharynx)

Causative Organism: <u>Borrelia</u> <u>vincentii</u>
　　　　　　　　　　　<u>Fusobacterium</u> <u>fusiform</u>

Characteristics of Organism (s):
　　　<u>Borrelia</u> <u>vincentii</u> -　a Spirochete
　　　　　　　　　　　　　　　Motile
　　　　　　　　　　　　　　　Non-spore forming
　　　　　　　　　　　　　　　Non-encapsulated
　　　　　　　　　　　　　　　also called
　　　　　　　　　　　　　　　<u>Treponema</u> <u>vincentii</u>

　　　<u>Fusobacterium</u> <u>fusiform</u>:

　　　　　　　　　　　　　　　Gram-negative - bacillus
　　　　　　　　　　　　　　　Non-motile
　　　　　　　　　　　　　　　Non-spore forming
　　　　　　　　　　　　　　　Non-encapsulated
　　　　　　　　　　　　　　　Facultative anaerobe
　　　　　　　　　　　　　　　also called
　　　　　　　　　　　　　　　<u>Leptotrichia</u> <u>bacillus</u>

Portal of Entry:
　　　Unknown

Predisposition:
　　　Age
　　　Fatigue/anxiety/stress
　　　Increase in corticosteroid
　　　Decrease lymphocytes

Clinical Symptoms:
　　　Pain
　　　Fever - 100°-101° F
　　　Interdental papillae - ulcerate/bleed
　　　　　　　　　　　　　　sloughing of tissue
　　　Fetid, metallic odor in mouth

175

Formation of pseudomembrane -
          clotted blood
          epithelial cells
          food
          lymphocytes
          bacteria
          (media for future growth)
Punched out lesions in gums
Bone destruction

Treatment:
    Teeth cleaning
    Antibiotics (rare)

Bacterial Diseases Acquired

via

Mucosal Membranes

Syphilis
Yaws
Pinta
Bejel
Gonorrhea
Granuloma Inguinale
Chancroid
Non-gonoccal urethritis
Acute Pyelonephritis
Cystitis
Gardnerellan Vaginitis

NAME OF DISEASE: Syphilis
OTHER NAME(S):   Leus, French disease, French pox

Causative Organism: <u>Treponema</u> <u>palladium</u>

Characteristics of Organism:
    Gram-negative spirochete
        tightly coiled (6-14 coils)
        axial filament in periplasmic space-
        composed of 3-6 fibrils
        well developed periplasmic space
        corkscrew motion
        5-15 micrometers by 0.25 micrometers
        fragile in environment - soaps
                        drying
                        temperature

    One Classical Scheme of Classification
        <u>T</u>. <u>palladium</u> <u>palladium</u> - syphilis
        <u>T</u>. <u>palladium</u> <u>endemicum</u> - bejel
        <u>T</u>. <u>palladium</u> <u>pertenue</u> - yaws
        <u>T</u>. <u>palladium</u> <u>carateum</u> - pinta
        (other schemes suggested)
    Strict growth conditions
        Minimal oxygen
        Highly specialized medium
        Anaerobic at 25°C - 2 weeks
        Generation time - 30 hours

Portal of Entry:
    Mucosal Membrane
    Congenital

Clinical Symptoms:
    3 stages
    Incubation - 10 to 90 days (average 3 weeks)
    Primary syphilis -   swollen area surrounding lymph nodes
                       Spirochetemia
                       Hard chancre - Hunterian
                       chancre - red

hard based
even-bordered
well-scribed
painless
glistening fluid -
filled center
highly infectious
Disappears - 3 to 12 weeks

Secondary syphilis -

4 weeks to 6 months later
Malaise
Lymphadenopathy
Thickened lymph node capsules
follicular hyperplasia in lymph
node
Increase in plasma cells in
lymph node
Fever
Flat, elevated, whitish-grey
patches of mucosa of
mouth - underneath
erythematous erosion
(snail tract ulcers)
condylomata lata

Luetic vasculitis -

endothelial cells
multiply - swell
walls of vessels thicken
(lymphocytes + fibrous
tissue)
Reduced lumen

Optic neuritis
CSF = decreased lymphocytes
          increased protein
Copper colored, annular, bilateral,
symmetrical rash
Pustular

Note -   ¼ patients recover - no symptoms, no
               antibodies

               ¼ show no symptoms but have antibodies

               ½ proceed to tertiary syphilis

Tertiary Syphilis
     Formation of gumma -   necrotizing ulcers
                                           granulomatous
                                           punched out appearance
                                           Perforation of body
                                           Effects skin, bone,
                                           liver, brain and heart
                                           Hypersensitivity reaction

     Argyll - Robertson pupil -

                                           adhesions
                                           fixed pupils
                                           irregular position
                                           atrophy of optic nerve

     CNS -   Meningitis
               destruction of cerebral cortex
                    Insanity
                    Deaf
                    Blind
                    Tabes dorsalis - slopping gait
                       (locomotorataxia)
                    Paresis - general paralysis
                       (dementia paralytica)
                    Tabetic crisis - referred pain
     Cardiac - leutic aortitis
               Aortic aneurysm

Osteoarthritis

Congenital
     Transferred after 4th month
     abortion

congenital syphilis -   Clutton's joints
                               Hutchinson teeth
                                (notched)
                               Moon's molars
                               Saddle nose
                               Sabre skins
                               Corneal inflammation
                               8th cranial nerve
                                deafness
                               Hepatic lobiatum - liver
                                parenchyma separated from
                                fibrous tissue
                               Pneumonic alba - fibrotic
                                inflammation - effects
                                adequate expansion
                                and aeration

Diagnosis:
   Microscopic -   Silver stains/negative stains
                    Dark field microscopy

   Serology -   Screening Tests - Floccillation tests
                       VDRL
                       PCT
                       USR
                       RPR
                       STS
                       Complement fixation
                       Kolmer
                       Wassermann
                    Others -
                       Eagle
                       Hinton
                       Mazzini
                       Reiter protein complement fixation
                        (RPCF)
                       Kahn
                       T. palladium complement - fixation (TPCF)

Specific Tests
　　Treponema paradium immobilization (TPI)
　　Preponema palladium adherence (TPA)
　　Imunnofluorenscense (FTA - ABS)
　　T. palladium microhemaglutination assay (MHATP)

Treatment:

　　Penicillin - large dose, long acting
　　Allergic - tetracycline
　　Pregnant, allergic - erythromycin
　　Doxycycline (Vibramycin)

NAME OF DISEASE: Yaws
OTHER NAMES(S):   Skerljeva, dishuchwa, njovera,
siti, frambesia, bouda, buba, pian
patela, frambesia tropica

Causative Organism: <u>Treponema</u> <u>pertenue</u>
<u>T</u>. <u>palladium</u> <u>perternue</u>

Characteristics of Organism:
  See Syphilis

Portal of Entry:
  Direct contact

Clinical Symptoms:
  Initial lesion -   "mother yaw"
                    raspberry like
  Develops -   large raspberry like excrescences
                    on soles of feet
                    painful papillomas
                    walk on side of foot

  Final stage -   Destruction of bone, cartilage, skin
                      Periostitis - tibia - saber
                    shins like syphilis
                    "boomerang legs"

  Dermal papilla -   hyperemic
                    edematous
                    plasma cells and neutrophils
                    predominate

  No effect on vascular system

Diagnosis:
  See Syphilis

Treatment:
  Long-acting penicillin
  one dose

NAME OF DISEASE   Pinta
OTHER NAME(S):   mal de pinto, larvate

Causative Organism: <u>Treponema</u> <u>carateum</u>
                        <u>T</u>. <u>palladium</u> <u>caratcium</u>

Characteristics of Organism:
    See syphilis

Portal of Entry:
    Direct contact
    possibly flies

Clinical Symptoms:
    Initial lesion -   flat, irregular margins
                            dry scaly infection - hands,
                                feet, scalp
                            Mottled (pigmented) skin

    Secondary lesions -   Copper to blue to white colored
                            becomes hypopigmented
                            Minimal involvement other systems
                            5-18 months - pale-pink macules
                            (pintids) - hyperkeratotic, depigmented

Diagnosis:
    See Syphilis

Treatment:
    Penicillin

NAME OF DISEASE: Bejel

Causative Organism: <u>Treponema</u> <u>endemic</u>
                        <u>Treponema</u> <u>palladium</u> <u>endemic</u>

Characteristics of Organism:
    See Syphilis

Portal of Entry:
    Direct contact

Clinical Symptoms:
    Lesions on breast - suckling mothers
    Secondary lesions in mouth like in syphilis
        Lesions of perineum / bone
        Gummas may form on breasts
        Spirochetes epidermal - neutrophils
            plasma cells -
            predominate

NAME OF DISEASE: Gonorrhea
OTHER NAMES(S):   Clap, strain, drip

Causative Organism: <u>Neisseria</u> <u>gonorrhea</u>

Characteristics of Organism:
    Gram-negative -   diplococci
                     kidney-bean shaped
                     look like donut

    Facultative anaerobe
    Ferments glucose - acid/no gas
    Non-motile
    Non-spore forming
    Non-encapsulated
    Sensitive to environment
    Pili - attachment
           Protease to digest IgA
           Virulence Factor
    Grows in leucocytes

Portal of Entry:
    Mucosal Membrane
    In male -   painful urination - urethritis dysuria
              Maeoprurlent discharge - yellowish
    Disseminated - bacteremia
              joint pain - arthritis
              fever
              skin lesions, pustular, hemorrhagic
                necrotic lesions

    In female -   symptoms rare
               pain lower abdomen

      Vulvovaginitis -   pre-pubescent mucosa, less keratin
                    painful urination
                    redness/edema
                    discharge
                    perianal soreness/discomfort on defecation

186

Gonococcal ophthalmia (Opthlmia neonatorum)
    Conjunctivitis in newborns
    Copious yellowish pus
    Untreated leads to blindness
    Broad - spectrum antibiotic

Course of Disease
    Attach via pili onto mucosa
    enveloped by microvilli
    become intracellular parasites
        (in leucocytes)
    Immune system like effect

Complications:
    In male -   conjunctivitis
                   proctitis
                   septicemia
                   sterility
                   urethral closure
                   epididymitis

    In female -   salpingitis
                   sterility
                   scarring of lymphaticus in pelvis - tight inflexible
                   tissue - "frozen pelvis"
                   PID

Diagnosis:

    Microscopic -   Leucocytes with diplococci
                               Specimen - pus

    Cultural -   Urethral, vaginal, rectal,
                           oral swabs
                           Media -chocolate
                               Thayer - Martin

    Serology -   ELISA
                          Monoclonal antibodies
                          Agglutination

187

Special techniques -   calorimetric techniques
(results in 10 minutes)
Oxidase test

Treatment:
    Long acting penicillin
    Resistant strains - spectinomycin
    allergic - tetracycline

Epidemiology
    Number one infectious disease with 2,000,000 to 4,000,000
    cases per year

NAME OF DISEASE: Granuloma inquinale
OTHER NAME(S):   Granuloma venereum

Causative Organism: <u>Calymmatobacterium granulomatous</u>
                        or <u>Donovani</u> <u>granlomatis</u>

Characteristics of Organism:
    Gram-negative pleomorphic bacillus
    Non-motile
    Non-spore forming
    Encapsulated
    Grows in egg yolk medias

Portal of Entry:
    Mucosal membrane

Clinical Symptoms:
    Incubation 1 to 6 months (iberia 2-4 weeks)
    Moist papules on genitals
    Painless
    Purple
    Ulcerates
    Reginal lymphadenopathy - rare

Diagnosis:

    Microscopic -   Smears from lesions
                Organism (safety-pin effect) in Monocytes

Treatment:
    Gentamicin
    Chloramphenicol
    also tetracycline, streptomycin

NAME OF DISEASE: Chancroid
OTHER NAME(S):   Soft chancre

Causative Organism: <u>Haemophilus</u> <u>ducreyi</u>
                         (Ducrey's Bacillus)

Characteristics of Organism:
    Gram-negative bacillus
    Non-motile
    Non-spore forming
    Cultured on blood agar
               defibrinated rabbit's blood

Portal of Entry:

Mucosal Membrane

Clinical Symptoms:
    Macular lesion changes to papuler
    To ragged, punched-out ulcer
        small, elevated
        soft-based, ragged-edged
        painful
        gray base
    Lymphadenopathy - supportive, unilateral
    Buboes - eruptive

Complications:
    Deep scars

Treatment:
    Erythromycin
    Trimethoprim - sulfamethoxazole

NAME OF DISEASE: Non-gonoccal urethritis
OTHER NAME(S):   NGU, Gonorcoccel like urethritis

Causative Organism: <u>Mima</u> <u>polymorpha</u>

Characteristics of Organism:
   Gram-negative, bacillus
   Bipolar staining
   Oxidase negative
   Non-motile
   Non-spore former
   Non-encapsulated

Portal of Entry:
   Mucous membrane

Clinical Symptoms:
   See gonorrhea

Diagnosis:
   Serology -   To distinguish from gonorrhea

Treatment:
   Streptomycin
   Spectinomycin

NAME OF DISEASE: Acute Pyelonephritis
Causative Organism: E. coli, Enterobacter aerogenous
    Proteus sp., Pseudomonas
    aeruginosa, staphylococcus,
    S. pyogenes

Portal of Entry:
   Hematogenous

Clinical Symptoms:
   Back pain
   Chill/slight fever
   Anorexia
   Cloudy urine (more than 100,000 CFU)
   Burning urination
   Micro abscesses
   Inflammation of renal parenchyma

Treatment:
   Nitrofurantoin
   Sulfonamides
   Tremithoprim
   Quinolones

NAME OF DISEASE: Cystitis
OTHER NAMES(S):   "Honeymoon" cystitis

Causative Organism(s):   <u>E.coli</u>, <u>P. vulgaris</u>
                            <u>P.aeruginosa</u>
                            coagulase-negative-
                            <u>S. saprophyticus</u>

Portal of Entry:
    Self introduction

Clinical Symptoms:
    Intercourse
    Painful micturition
    Dysuria
    Pyrouria - burning urination
    Hematuria
    Leucocytes in urine

Treatment:
    Nitrofurantoin
    Gantrisin (sulf, soxazule)
    Ampicillin

NAME OF DISEASE: Gardnerellan vaginitis
Causative Organism: Garnerella vaginitis

Characteristics of Organism:
    Gram-negative, bacillus
    Grows ph 5-6
    Non-motile
    Non-spore forming
    Course -   Lactobacillus decrease
                    Bacteroides increase
                    help create environment

Clinical Symptoms:
    In female -   Frothy vaginal discharge
                  malodorous

    In male -   Balanitis
                  lesions on penis

Diagnosis:
    Microscopic - Vaginal swab
                  Clue cells - epithelial cells
                          with bacilli inside

Treatment:
    metronidazole (Flagl)

BACTERIAL DISEASES

via

GASTRO-INTESTINAL ROUTE

Typhoid Fever
Paratyphoid Fever
Salmonellosis
Shigellosis
Cholera
Staphylococcal Food Poisoning
Perfringen Food Poisoning
Botulism
Vibrio Parahaemotypticus Enteritis
Brucellosis
Leptospirosis
Campylobacter Food Poisoning
E. Coli Food/Water Poisoning
Yersiniosis
Bacillus Gastroenteritis
Antibiotic Associated Colitis

NAME OF DISEASE: Typhoid Fever

Causative Organism: <u>Salmonella</u> <u>thyphosa</u>

Characteristics of Organism:
      Gram-negative bacillus
      Motile
      Non-spore forming
      Encapsulated - 3 antigens
            O - antigen - cellular
            H - antigen - flagellar
            V_1 - antigen - capsular
      Ferments - glucose (possibly with gas) not lactose
      Hydrogen sulfide positive
      Urease negative
      Citrate negative
      Acid - resistant
      Survives in environment
      Freeze - resistant
      Classed into 3 species and over 1800 serotypes in
           Kaufman-White scheme

Portal of entry:
      Gastro-intestinal route
      Reservoir - Man
      High infective dose
      Urine from patients with pyelonephritis

Clinical Symptoms:
      Incubation - 10 to 14 days
      5 stages -
            Active invasion/bacteremia - 1 week
            Fatigue stage - about 1 week
            Lytic stage - 1 week
            Convalescence - many weeks
      Fever - 104°F, increases over 3 day - stepwise spiking in
           afternoon
      Abdominal tenderness
      Diarrhea/constipation - bleeding
      Vomiting

Pink to red maculas on abdomen
Edematous, infiltrated with histiocytes
Splenomegaly
Slow pulse
Lymphocytopenia

Course of Disease:
    Survives acidity of stomach
    Attach to villi of small intestines
    Multiply and invade mucosa
    Ulcerate
    To lymphoid follicles/peyer's patches
    Phagocytized, but live and multiplying in phagocytes
    Focal granulomas on liver
    Go to liver, kidney, gall bladder (may have to be removed)
    Release to RES - to thoracic duct
    Typhoid nodules in organs composed of macrophages,
            phagocytized bacteria, RBC, degenerated WBC's
    Bacteremia
    Untreated - last about a month
                    15 - 20 % mortality
    Cholecystitis
    Thrombophlebitis

Complications:
    Peritonitis - perforation of bowel
    Meningitis - ring hemorrhage (microthrombi)
    Pneumonia (interstitial)
    Complications of toxemia -
            faulty liver
            flabby heart (dilation of ventricles)
            vacuolization of cardiac myocytes
            cardiac arrhythmia
            proximal tubular epithelium damage in kidney
            degeneration of skeletal muscle

197

Diagnosis:

    Specimens -   stool   urine

                    blood   bone marrow

    Serology -   Widal Test

                   ELISA Test

                   DNA probe

    Cultural -   Medias - Bismuth sulfite

                             Salmonella - shigella

                             EMB agar

                             Maconkey

                             Hektoen

                             Triple sugar

                             Kliger's Iron agar

Special Tests:

    IMViC - Test for

                    Indole production

                    acid fermentation

                    Voges - Proskauer test

                    citrate utilization

    IMVIC combined with other tests such as motility, H_2S, gelatinase urease, etc. - used in two kits

                    Enterotube

                    API/20E

Treatment:

    Chloramphenicol + tetracycline

    2 + weeks

    or - Amoxicillin

    or - Tremethoprim - sulfamethoxazole

    or - Ceftriaxone

Epidemiology:

    400-600 cases/year

NAME OF DISEASE: Paratyphoid Fever

Causative Organism: <u>Salmonella</u> <u>enteritidis</u>
                                    (<u>Salmonella</u> <u>paratyphi</u>)

Characteristics of Organism:
        See Typhoid Fever

Portal of Entry: Gastro-intestinal

Clinical Symptoms:
        Shorter course than typhoid
        Less severe than typhoid
        Lower mortality rate
        Transient diarrhea
        Fever

Epidemiology:
        Paratyphi A = <u>S.</u> <u>paratyphi</u>
        Paratyphi B = <u>S.</u> <u>schottmuelleri</u>
        Paratyphi C = <u>S.</u> <u>hirschfeldii</u>

NAME OF DISEASE: Salmonellosis
OTHER NAME(S):   Salmonellan gastroenteritis,
                   "food-poisoning"

Causative Organism: <u>Salmonella</u> <u>enteritidis</u>

Characteristics of Organism:
        See typhoid fever

Portal of Entry: Gastro-intestinal

Symptoms:
                Incubation - 6 - 36 hours
                Fever vis endotoxin
                Diarrhea (bloody in infants)
                Nausea/vomiting
                Dizziness

Diagnosis:
                ELISA
                DNA probe

Treatment:
                antibiotics only to very young and old
                self-limiting

Epidemiology:
        Common sources - Poultry/eggs
                          Pets - dogs/cats
                                  turtles, chicks, bunnies
                          Rats/mice
                          Unclorinated water
                          Food dyes like carmine red made of
                                  crushed insect abdomens

Prevention:

Proper cooking of poultry (145°-160°)
Proper handling after cooking (refrigeration)
Proper refrigeration
Inspection of food handlers, handwashing (under finger nail)
Care with transport/storage of poultry shellfish, eggs
Personal hygiene
Chlorination

Over 40,000 cases/year and this is but the tip

NAME OF DISEASE: Shigellosis
OTHER NAME(S):   bacillary dysentery,
        "gay-bowel syndrome"

Causative Organism: <u>Shigella</u> <u>dysenteriae</u>
        (shiga's bacillus)
        <u>S</u>. <u>sonnei</u>
        <u>S</u>. <u>flexneri</u>
        <u>S</u>. <u>boydii</u>

Characteristics of Organism:
    Gram-negative bacillus
    Mon-motile
    Non-spore forming
    Non-encapsulated
    Does not survive out of stool well
        sensitive to - heat
                    drying
                    disinfectants
    No H_2S
    No urease

Portal of Entry:
    Gastro-intestinal
    Anal intercourse
    Low infective dose

Clinical Symptoms:
    Incubation - 48 hours
    Fever (only children) - endotoxin
    Exotoxin effects adenyl cyclase of intestinal wall
    Results in diarrhea
    Gripping pain (adults)
    Tenesmus
    Diarrhea contains blood, mucous and pus (red currant jelly
        stools)
    Rectal burning
    Loss of water

No perforation of bowel
Mucosa - edematous
        hyperemia
        ulceration - bowel-covered,   dirty-yellow
           pseudomembrane

Course of disease:
    Organism to epithelium of large intestine
    Goes to submucosa
    Ulcers lesions
    Inflammation

Complications:
    Loss of fluid: leads protein deficiency, lack of B_{12}
                     (anemia), electrolytes
    Exotoxin: (shiga's toxin): is a neurotoxin, affects blood
                           vessels, neurological symptoms

Diagnosis: see Typhoid Fever
             Specimens - Rectal swabs
             Serology - agglutination
             Special Tests - API 20E/EMB

Treatment:
    Replace fluids
    Balance of electrolytes
    Multiple Drug Resistant testing
        Possibilities - ampicillin
                           Nalidixic acid
                           Trimethoprim - sulfamethoxazole

Epidemiology:
    about 20,000 cases/year
    no animal reservoir
    affects mainly young (½ of cases)
    related to confined populations

NAME OF DISEASE: Cholera
OTHER NAME(S):   Asiatic cholera

Causative Organism: <u>Vibrio chlorae</u>
        (<u>Vibrio comma</u>)

Characteristics of Organism:
    Gram negative - curved bacillus
    Motile - polar flagella
        moves in helical path with wobble darting motion
    Facultative anaerobe
    Fermentation - acids/no gas
    2 bio types -   classic (100 serotypes)
            El Tor - produces hemolysins
    Killed by heat, acid
    Virulence factors - colicins
            mucinase
            neuraminidase
            enterotoxin - choleragen
            (increases cAMP production)
    Medias - Alkaline peptone broth
        Monsur
        TCBS agar (thiosulfate, citrate, bile salts

Portal of Entry: Gastro-intestinal route
        Fecal-Oral route
        High infective dose - due to acidity of
            stomach

Clinical Symptoms:
    Incubation - hours to 5 days
    Severe abdominal pain
    Severe vomiting
    Painless, profuse, watery diarrhea with flecks of mucous
        ("rice-water stools")
    Fluid loss - 20-25 liters/day
    Thirst

Wrinkled skin
Acidosis
Concentration of blood elements
    lack of oxygen to brain
Tachycardia/tachypnea
Lack of bowel sounds
Hypochloremia
Oliguria or complete renal shut down
Muscle cramps due to renal loss
Weak pulse

Course of Disease:
    Ingestion to small intestine (duodenum-jejunum)
    Multiply
    Infiltrate mucosal cells and into-exocrine ducts
    No penetration of mucosa
    Release toxins
    Stimulate cAMP
    Release of isotonic solution , electrolytes, mucous

Complications: Neurological
                 Anemia

Diagnosis:
    Microscopic - Direct dark-field microscopy
    Cultural - Cholera Red Test
            (Conversion of nitrate to nitrite)
    Serology -   agglutination
                 phage typing

Tetracycline: Replace fluids
                 IV
                 Oral dehydrant - water, glucose - 20 grams, NaCl
                   - 4.2 grams, KCl - 1.8 grams, $NaHCO_3$ - 4.0
                   trams per liter
                 Reduces mortality from 55% to almost 0%
                 Tetracycline

205

Epidemiology:
Vaccine of limited value

3 serotypes - A = Inaba
B = Ogawa
C = Hikojima

<u>V. vulnufieus</u> - a halophilic vibrio infects open wounds
leads to - cellulitis
septicemia
Portal entry - food

206

NOTES:

NAME OF DISEASE: Staphylococcal Food Poisoning

Causative Organism: <u>Staphylococcus</u> <u>aueus</u>

Characteristics of Organism:
    See staphylococcal pneumonia

    Enterotoxin produce - moderate heat stable
        withstands 100°C for ½ hour
    5 enterotoxins - A through E

Portal of Entry: Gastro-intestinal

Clinical Symptoms:
    Incubation - 1 to 6 hours
    Nausea/vomiting (toxin stimulates vagus nerve)
    Cramps,, abdominal
    Diarrhea
    No fever
    Bluish tinge to skin
    Lasts 18-24 hours

Diagnosis:
    Difficult, other than clinical picture
    Serology for enterotoxin - gel diffusion

Treatment:
    Rare

Epidemiology:
    2nd most common food poisoning in United States
    Usual sources - Bakery goods - custards and creams
                     Cured, processed meats (grow well in salt)
                     Fish
                     Diary products
    Prevention -   Care in food handling
                     Personal hygiene
                     Refrigeration

NOTES:

NAME OF DISEASE: Perfringen Food Poisoning

Causative Organism: <u>Clostridia</u> <u>perfringens</u>

Characteristics of Organism:
        Gram-positive bacillus
        Strict anaerobe (less so
        than <u>S.</u> <u>botulinum</u>)
        Non-encapsulated
        Spore-forming
        Non-motile
        Enterotoxin - 6 types
        (A-F)

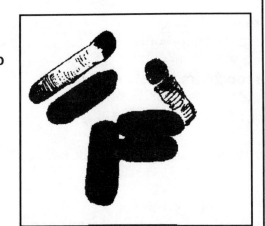
Clostridia perfrigens

Portal of Entry:
  Gastro-intestinal - ingestion

Clinical Symptoms:
        Incubation - 8-24 hours
        Similar to staphylococcal food poisoning
        Lasts 6-12 hours

Diagnosis:
        Culture - Fluid thioglycollate broth
                   Motility - nitrate media
                   Other medias - SPS agar-
                                  Sulfite-polymyxin-
                                  Sulfadiazine
                                  TSA agar-
                                  Tryptone - sulfite - neomycin

Treatment: Symptomatic -
            Possible - penicillin, antitoxin (rare)

208

NAME OF DISEASE: Botulism
OTHER NAME(S): "Sausage" disease

Causative Organism: <u>Clostridium</u>
<u>botulinum</u>

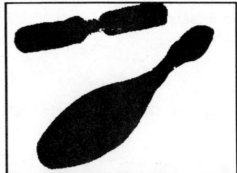
<u>Clostridium</u> <u>botulinum</u>

Characteristics of Organism:
Gram-positive, bacillus,
singly or pairs
Strict anaerobe
Motile - peritrichous
flagella
Spore-forming
Neurotoxins: via
lysogenic
conversion
6-8 toxins - A-H
4 cause disease in men
Blocks acetylcholine
Heat sensitive -
destroyed 10 min at 100°C
Type A- most toxic
absorbed
through skin
breaks down
protein
notable
ammonia odor
if high protein
environment
Type B- mortality
25% untreated
Type E- Found in
marine and
lake seafood
no smell
produced
even in
refrigeration

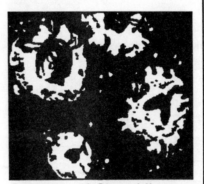
Colonies of <u>Clostridium</u>
<u>botulinum</u>

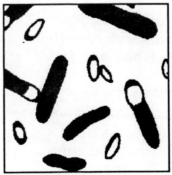
<u>Clostridia</u> <u>botulinum</u>

Six antigenic types - A through F
Fermentation - acid/gas production

Portal of Entry: Gastro-intestinal -
                               ingestion

Course of Disease:
        Resistant to stomach acid
        Absorbed into blood from
        intestines
        To cholinergic nerve endings at
        myoneural junctions
        Bind at membrane receptors
        (gangliosides)
        Inhibits release of acetylcholine
        Muscles paralyzed in relaxed position

Clinical Symptoms:
        Incubation - 12-38 hours
        Speech problems (diphonia)
        Blurry/double vision (diplopia)
        Weakness/dizziness
        Dysphagia
        Dry mouth
        Diarrhea/vomiting
        Dysarthria
        Paralysis of - urinary bladder
                               respiratory system - death
                               cardiac system - death

Diagnosis:
        In vivo tests - mice inoculation
        Serology - Toxin precipitation
        Physiology - electromyogram

Treatment:
       Antitoxin - type specific
              Initially trivalent type A,B,E
              Then monovalent on determination
       Respirator
       Gastro-intestinal evacuation
       Note: once toxin attaches to junction difficult to dissociate

Epidemiology:
       Other forms
              Wound botulism -
                     Portal of Entry - break in skin
                     Symptoms -
                            descending paralysis along cranial nerves
              Infant botulism - "Floppy-body" syndrome
                     Usually associated with honey
                     Symptoms - lethargic
                            lack of suckling/swallow
                            constipation
                            paralysis - hand, neck, arms, back
                            death - respiratory paralysis

NAME OF DISEASE: Vibrio parahaemotypticus enteritis

Causative Organism: <u>Vibrio</u> <u>parahaemolyticus</u>

Characteristics of Organism:
        Gram-negative - curved rod
        Motile - polar flagella
        Halophilic - differs from <u>V. cholerae</u>
        Non-Fermentative
        Soluble hemolysin (goat's blood)
        Grows up to temperatures of 42°C
        Generation time - 10 min.

Portal of Entry:
        Gastro-intestinal - Contaminated seafood

Clinical Symptoms:
        Incubation less than 24 hours
        Burning sensation - stomach
        Abdominal pain/cramping
        Explosive diarrhea/vomiting
                (similar to cholera)
        Recovery - few days

Diagnosis:
        Rectal swabs grown on
        TCBS agar (thiosulfate, nitrate, bile salts)
        BTB - teepol agar - (Bromothymol blue-)
        35°C - 18/24 hours
        Blue - green colonies

Treatment: If necessary
            Tetracycline
            Chloramphenicol
            Penicillin

Epidemiology:

      Common food poisoning in Japan
      From chitinous skeletons of crustaceans
      Particularly harvested after "upwelling"
      Cutaneous form of disease -   through breaks in skin -
                                     swimmers cuts/abrasions
                                     from shells

213

NAME OF DISEASE: Brucellosis
OTHER NAME(S):   Undulating Fever, Malta Fever,
                    Bang's Disease, Goat Fever,
                    Rio Grande Fever

Causative Organism: various species of <u>Brucella</u>

Characteristics of Organism:
        Gram-negative - small
                bacillus
        Non-motile
        Non-spore forming
        Non-encapsulated/
            encapsulated
        Slow growing
        Strict pathogen
        Stable in environments
        Survives in
            macrophages
        Complex media required
        Usual species involved
                <u>B. abortus</u> - cow
                <u>B. suis</u> - pig
                <u>B. melitensis</u> - goat
                <u>B. canis</u> - dog
        Zoonoses - from animals

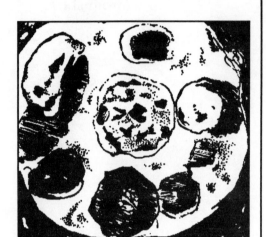

<u>Brucella</u> in large vacoule in a phagocyte

Portal of Entry: Gastro-intestinal
                  Venereally

Course of Disease:
        Enters mucosa of small intestines
        To neutrophils - release bacteria
        To RES, kidney

214

Clinical Symptoms:

> Incubation - 5 to 35 days
> 3 types -
>> 1. Acute malignant - Flu-like
>>> high fever/chills
>>> fluctuating fever - high afternoon, low night
>>> night sweats
>>> prostration
>>> somatic pain
>>> lymphadenopathy
>>> liver/spleen involvement
>>> jaundiced
>> 2. Recurrent - wavelike relapse
>>> decrease in severity
>> 3. Chronic (intermittent)
>>> gradual increase in malaise
>>> weight loss
>>> fever mild
>>> depression/fatigue
>>> abscesses, groin, gonads, kidney

B. suis enters even through unbroken skin, characterized by necrotic abbscesses

Complications:

> Spondylitis
> Orchitis
> Subacvite endocarditis
> learning/visual impairment
> hemiplegic/ataxia
> osteomyelitis
> pyelonephritis
> abortion

Diagnosis:

> Specimen -   blood
> Cultural -   Enriched media
>   microaerophilic incubation

Serology -   agglulication
              phage-typing
              fluorescent antibody test
              ELISA
Skin -   Brucellergen skin test

Treatment:
    Tetracycline/streptomycin
    + Cortieosteroids (severe cases)

NAME OF DISEASE: Leptospirosis
OTHER NAME(S):   Weil's Disease, spirochetal jaundice

Causative Organism: <u>Leptospira</u> <u>interrogans</u>,
                                    serotypes - <u>icterohemorrhagica</u>
                                                      <u>canicola</u>
                                                      <u>pomona</u>

Characteristics of Organism:
        Spirochete (leptospiral)
        4 - 20 micrometers by 0.1 micrometers
        Motile
        Tightly-coiled
        Hooked or looped ends
        Easily killed with heat, drying, disinfectant
        Stains best with silver impregnation or Giemsa
        Media -   must contain serum such as 10% heat incubated
                         rabbit serum
                   Stuart's media
                   Fletcher's media
                   Korthof's media
                   also - fertile hen's egg

Portal of Entry: Gastro-intestinal-ingestion
                         Mucosal membranes

Clinical Symptoms:
        Incubation - average 50 days
        2 phases -
                1. Leptospironemic phase
                        (in blood - CSF)
                        High fever/chills
                        headache
                        muscleache/tenderness
                        conjunctivitis/suffusion
                        vomiting - blackish
                2. Immune stage - Weil's Disease
                        increased IgM
                        myalgia
                        abdominal pain
                        fever

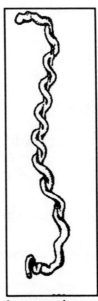

<u>Leptospira</u>
<u>interrogans</u>

hepatic failure stained with bile/jaundice
kidney failure - pus in urine
hemorrhages of organs
pulmonary edema
liver -   erythrophagocytosis
           neutrophilic infiltration of sinusoids
           necrosis of hepatocytes
kidney -   swelling of tubular epithelium,
           necrosis

Diagnosis:
Serology -   slide agglutination
              (microagglutination)
              complement - fixation
              immune - adherence
              fluorescent antibody
Microscopy - Early in disease - dark-field microscopy
              (blood or urine)

Treatment: Penicillin

Epidemiology:
100-150 cases/year

Serotypes associated with - canicola - dogs
                            icterohemorrhagicum - rats
                            pomona - cattle/pigs

Vaccine for dogs, organism transmitted by urine

Patient isolation warranted - blood, urine

NAME OF DISEASE: Campylobacteran gastroenteritis

Causative Organism: <u>Campylobacter</u> <u>jejuni</u>
                        also <u>C-fetus</u>

Characteristics of Organism:
        Gram-negative, curved spirillum
        Non-spore forming
        Non-encapsulated
        Motile - flagellar - polar
        Microaerophilic
        Enterotoxin - EJT
        (campylobacter jejunal toxins)

Portal of Entry:
        Gastro-intestinal - ingestion

Clinical Symptoms:
        Incubation 1-7 days
        Abdominal pains
        Diarrhea
        Nausea/vomiting
        Fever
        Myalgia
        Malodorous, bloody stools
        Inflammation - jejunum to anus
                (ulcer-crypt abbesses)
        Small intestines - edematous
                            hyperemic
                            infiltration of neutrophils
                            lymphocytes, plasma cells

Treatment:
        Rehydration
        Quinolones
        Erythromycin
        Aminoglycosides
        Chloramphenicol

Epidemiology:
    Source - underdone chicken
               non-hygienic chicken (non-chlorinated water in
                      processing)
               unpasteurized milk

NAME OF DISEASE: <u>E. coli</u> gastroenteritis
OTHER NAME(S):   Traveler's diarrhea, Montezuma's revenge,
                  Delhi belly

Causative Organism: <u>Escherichia</u> <u>coli</u>

Characteristics of Organism:
        Gram-negative, bacillus
        Non-spore-former
        Pili
        Encapsulated
        Indole-positive
        Methyl - red-positive
        Voges - Proskauer-negative
        Citrate - negative
        Lactose fermented - acid/gas
        Motile/non-motile
        Facultative anerole

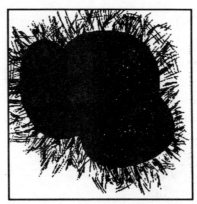
Enterpetohogenic <u>E. coli</u>

Various types -
        Enterotoxigenic E. coli (ETEC)
                2 toxins - heat labile
                            activates cAMP
                            heat stable
                            impairs sodium, chlorides absorption
                            reduction of motility of intestines
                            attaches via pili
                            diarrheal diseases
                            lysogenic conversion
        Enteroinvasive E. coli (EIEC)
                Shigellosis-like disease
                Local tissue destruction
                Necrosis of mucosa-sloughing
                Blood in stools/neutrophisis
        Enterohemorrhegic E. coli (EHEC)
                Reservoir cattle
                Hemorrhagic colitis
                Copious blood
                No fever

Enteroadhesive E. coli (EAEC)
        Plasmid mediated
        Pili attachment
        Mechanism unknown

Portal of Entry:
    Gastro-Intestinal

Clinical Symptoms:
    Epidemic   Neonatal diarrhea
                  Severe diarrhea (cholera-like)
                  Yellow to green
                  Cyanosis
                  Convulsions
                  Dehydration
                  Jaundice
                  Lethargic
                  Via somatic antigens
    Traveler's Diarrhea
                  Cramps
                  Pus
                  Bloody stools
                  Due to enterotoxin

Diagnosis:
    Cultural - EMB agar
                  hektoen agar
    Chemical - IMViC
                  Enterotube
                  API/2OE

Treatment:
    Rare
    Kaolin, pectin -   give diarrheal relief, but bacteria retain and grow
    Better - Peptobismal -   a bismuth - salicylic mixture

NAME OF DISEASE: Yersinial gastroenteritis

Causative Organism: <u>Yersinina</u> <u>enterocolitica</u>
                     <u>Y.</u> <u>pseudotuberculosis</u> in infected animals

Characteristics of Organism:
    Gram-negative - bacillus
    Free-living
    Grows in refrigerator
    Motile at 4∘C, not at 37∘C
    Produces enterotoxin

Portal of Entry: Gastro-intestinal
                  Source - frequently "chitterlings"

Course of Disease:
    Multiply in ileum
    Invade mucosa
    Go to Peyer's patches -   ulceration
                              necrosis
    To mesenteric lymph node

    Pseudo tuberculosis form to ileocecum
        to lymph nodes
        to liver spleen
        course granulomas

223

NAME OF DISEASE: Bacillus gastroenteritis

Causative Organism: <u>Bacillus</u> <u>cereus</u>

Clinical Symptoms:
      Nausea/vomiting
      Abdominal cramps
      Diarrhea
      via enterotoxin

Epidemiology:
      Air/dustborne
      Found in cooked foods - rice, potatoes, meat
      Organism survives short heating-spores
          cooling - vegetative cells grow

NAME OF DISEASE: Antibiotic associated colitis

Causative Organism: <u>Clostridia</u> <u>difficile</u>

Characteristics of Organism:
    see botulism

Clinical Symptoms:
    When other types of bacteria destroyed by antibiotics if
        cause superinfection
    Diarrhea - late in disease
    Cramps
    Fever
    Leucocytosis
    Colonic inflammation
    Sloughing of mucosal membrane
    Local perforation

Treatment:
    Remove antibiotics
    If not effective use vancomycin

BACTERIAL DISEASES

via

ARTHROPOD BITES

Bubonic Plague
Tularemia
Pasteurellosis
Bartonellosis
Relapsing Fever

NAME OF DISEASE: Bubonic Plague
OTHER NAME(S):   Plague, "Black death"

Causative Organism: <u>Yersinia</u> <u>pestis</u>
        was called <u>Pasteurella</u> <u>pestis</u>

Characteristics of Organism:
        Gram-negative, coccobacillus
        Safety-pin staining effect
        Non-motile
        Non-spore forming
        Facultative anaerobe
        Ferments -   glucose
                    levulose
                    maltose
                    mannitol
                    acid/no gas
        Slow growing, best at 30°C
        Can grow in phagocytes
        Virulence factors - capsule/envelop protein
                            coagulase
                            endotoxin
                            murine toxin - blocks esophagus of vector, ravished, spreads disease more quickly by vector trying to get food
                        causes: swelling
                               necrosis
                               electrolyte imbalance

Portal of Entry: Break in skin
        Vector - flea (<u>Xenophyllus</u>, <u>Pulex</u>)
        Reservoir - rats
        also, cat scratches
        Skinning animals (indirect)

Clinical Symptoms:

3 forms
1. Bubonic
Incubation - 2 to 6 days
Entrance - frequently legs
To inguinale lymph nodes - painful
Swelling
Fever
Rapid respiration
Rapid pulse
Lymph nodes become inflamed, suppurative buboes
Become hemorrhagic, necrotic
Turn black (petechial ecchymoses)
Untreated - mortality 60-75% in days
Treated - mortality 20-25%

2. Septicemic
Directly in blood stream, little or no lymph node involvement
Massive tissue damage
Fever
Prostration
Meningitis
Disseminated intravascular coagulation
Circulatory stagnation
Subcutaneous hemorrhagic
Purpura
Gangrene
Pleural effusion
Pericarditis
Untreated - mortality 100%
Treated - mortality 20-29%

3. Pneumonic - See plague pneumonia

Diagnosis:
    Hematology - Increased WBC

    Cultural -   Specimens - blood
                                  sputum
                                  lymph node aspirates
                     Blood agar - grey viscous colonies

    Microscopic - Stains -   Wayson (methylene blue and
                               carbol fuchsin)

    Serology -   Phage-typing
                  Fluorescent antibody
                  4-fold titre increase

Treatment:
    Streptomycin
    Tetracycline
    (The longer treatment delayed, the less successful, don't
        wait for lab results)

Epidemiology:
    Sylvatic (campestral) plague -
        endemic southwest
        milder form - localized buboes
        risk group - hunters
        reservoir - wild rodents

    Plague is a zoonosis -
        an animal disease in which man gets in the way of harm

    Other terms -
        enzootic -   a disease endemic in animals
        epizootic -   a disease from animals to man

    Control -   Rat control
                 Flea control
               Vaccine - Haffkine's, limited use
                         Formaldehyde inactivated bacteria
                             grown on artificial media

NAME OF DISEASE: Tularemia
OTHER NAME(S):   Rabbit Fever, Deer Fly Fever,
                      O'Hara's Disease

Causative Organism: <u>Francisella</u> <u>tularensis</u>
                       used to be <u>Pasteurella</u> <u>tularensis</u>

Characteristics of Organism:
      Gram-negative, bacillus
         (small)
      Facultative anaerobe
      Non-motile
      Non-spore forming
      Non-encapsulated
      Grows in blood agar +
         cystine
      Two biovars -
         Type A - virulent
                   tick   is
                      vector
                   reservoir - rabbit
                   mortality - 5-30% untreated
         Type B - less virulent
                   wider distribution
                   mortality less than 1% even if untreated

<u>Francisella   tularensis</u>

Portal of Entry:
      Contact infected animal
      Tick, bite
      Contaminated water
      over 20 means of transmission

Clinical symptoms:
      Incubation- 3 to 10 days

         1. Ulceroglandular
             form - (skin)
             tender
             erythematous
             papule at point of entry

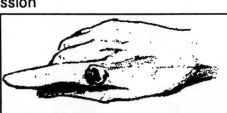

Tularemia

becomes tender pustule
ulcerates
to regional lymph nodes
enlarge
bacteremia
lymphadenopathy/splenomegaly (in a week)
possible to lungs - necrotic pneumonia
also endotoxin shock
headache - severe
fever - high
relapses frequent

2. Oculoglandular -
papule on conjunctiva
pustule
ulcerates
lymphadenopathy - head/neck
infection optic nerve
blindness

3. Bacteremia -
resembles typhoid
high fever
abdominal pain

Diagnosis:
Specimens -   aspirates lymph nodes

Serology -   antibody titre increase

Cultural -   on blood agar + cystine
colonies 4-7 days

Skin test -   Foshay's

When working with organism use hood - very low infective
dose (less than 50 organisms)

231

Treatment:
>   Streptomycin
>   Gentamicin
>
>   (Difficult due to fact organism is an intracellar parasite)

Epidemiology:
>   Steadily increasing by a factor of 10 over 50 years
>   About 200 cases/year

NAME OF DISEASE: Pasteurellosis

Causative Organism: <u>Pasteurella</u> <u>multicoida</u>

Characteristics of Organism:
      Gram-negative, coccobacillus
      Facultative anaerobe
      Ferments - glucose
        Acid/no gas
      Non-motile
      Non-spore forming
      Non-encapsulated
      Produces hydrogen sulfide

Portal of Entry:
      Arthropod bite
      Animal scratch

Clinical Symptoms:
      Rapid onset
      Marked pain/swelling at initial site
      Fever
      Lymphadenopathy
      Untreated leads to -   septicemia
                              pseudotuberculosis
                              pneumonia

Treatment:
      Penicillin
      Tetracycline

NAME OF DISEASE: Bartonellosis
OTHER NAME(S):   Carrion's Disease (Oroyo fever), Verruga peruana (peruviana)

Causative Organism: <u>Bartonella</u> <u>bacilliformis</u>

Characteristics of Organism:
    Gram-negative - coccobacillus
    Motile
    Non-spore forming
    Non-encapsulated
    Parasitizes RBC
    Grown in embryonated eggs

Portal of Entry:
    Break in skin
    Vector - sandfly (<u>Phlebotomus</u>)

Clinical Symptoms:
    Incubation - 14 to 21 days
    2 stages
        1. Oroyo fever - fever
                skeletal pain
                diarrhea/vomiting
                microcytic, hemolytic anemia
                lymphadenopathy
                hepatosplenomegaly
                untreated - mortality 40%
        2. Verruga Peruviana -

                benign wart-like lesions like
                    hemangiomas
                nodular lesions on joints-limit mobility
                mortality - untreated less than 5%

Verruga Peruana

Diagnosis:
    Cultural -   semisolid media with hemoglobin and rabbit serum
    Microscopic - Giemsa - reddest violet
                  Wright's - blue

NAME OF DISEASE: Relapsing Fever
OTHER NAME(S):   Tick Fever, Fowl-nest Fever,
                      Vagabond Fever, Cabin Fever, bilious
                      typhoid, borreliosis

Causative Organism: <u>Borrelia</u> <u>recurrentis</u> - louse-borne
                    <u>Borrelia</u> <u>duttonii</u> - tick borne
                    (also <u>B. turicatae</u>, <u>B. porberi</u> and <u>B. hermesil</u>)

Characteristics of Organism:
    Spirochete - 10 to 20 micrometers by 0.2 to 0.5
        micrometers
    Long loose spirals (4-30)
    30-40 periplasmic flagella
    Stain with aniline dyes
    Does not grow well on artificial medias -
                                Use Kelly's broth
                                Mice
                                Fertile hen's egg

Portal of Entry:
    Epidemic form - (<u>B. recurrentis</u>)
                    Lice's bodies crushed, rubbed in wound
    Endemic form - Vector tick

Clinical Symptoms:
    Incubation period - 3 to 10 days (average 7 days)
    High fever - 104°F
    Headache/muscleache
    Diarrhea/vomiting
    Lethargy
    Joint pain
    Hepatosplenomegaly
    Conjunctival hemorrhages
    Abdominal tenderness
    Rose spots
    Jaundice
    Pulse/respiration increased

In severe cases
      coma
      meningitis
      myocarditis
      liver failure, inflammation or sinusoids
      other organs - kidney
      cranial nerves
      spleen - microabcesses to neurosis
Untreated - mortality 5-40%

Can cross placenta

Fever lasts 5-9 days, then disappears for 7-10 days and
    repeats over and over, hence name. This is due to
    rapidly changing surface antigens.

Diagnosis:
    Specimens -   blood
    Microscopy - dark field
                stain Wright's or Giemsa
    Serology -   difficult with changing antigens
    Animal inoculation
    Hematology - increased WBC (lymphocytes)
                increased RBC sedimentation rate

Treatment:
    Tetracycline
    Penicillin
    Not to be given at height of disease because possibility of
      Jarisch-Herxheimer Reaction (JHR)

Epidemiology:
    Spriochote will give false positive syphilis test
    JHR - due to endotoxin
        fever
        joint pain
        delirium
        diarrhea
        coughing fits

Bacterial Diseases

via

Skin

Sodoku
Haverhill Fever
Anthrax
Gas Gangrene
Tetanus
Hansen's Disease
Pseudonomal Infections
Staphylococcal Infections
Erysipeloid

NAME OF DISEASE: Sodoku
OTHER NAME(S):   Rat Bite Fever

Causative Organism: <u>Spirillum</u> <u>minus</u>

Characteristics of Organism:
    Spirochete - 15 micrometers by 2 to 5 micrometers
    Rigid coils - 1-6
    Motile - Lophotrichous flagella
        1-7
    Non-spore forming
    Non-encapsulated

Portal of Entry:
    Rate Bite

Clinical Symptoms
    Primary -   Localized inflammation
        Headache
        Heals

    Secondary -   2-3 weeks later
        Lesions elsewhere - palms/soles
        Intermittent fever
        Inflammation lymph nodes
            (lymph adenitis)
        Red to dark purple rash
        Arthritis - possible
        Endocarditis

    Symptoms will disappear/relapse

Diagnosis:
    Specimens blood
    Microscopy -   Dark field
        Stain - Aniline dyes
Treatment:
    Penicillin
    (Not during height of infection - concern for Jarisch-Herxheimer Reaction)

238

NAME OF DISEASE: Haverhill Fever
OTHER NAME(S):   Rat bite fever

Causative organism: <u>Streptobacillus moniliformis</u>

Characteristics of Organism:
    Gram-negative - bacillus
    Aerobe
    Non-encapsulated
    Non-spore forming
    Non-motile

Portal of Entry:
    Rat bite
    Contaminate milk

Streptobacillus
moniliformis

Clinical Symptoms:

    Relapsing fever
    Red to purple rash
    Regional lymphadenitis
    Possible   arthritis
                endocarditis

Diagnosis:

    Specimens -   blood
                      joint aspirates

    Cultural -   media with blood and serum
                    small colonies
                    observe L-form
                    (cell wall defect)

Treatment:
    Penicillin

NAME OF DISEASE: Anthrax
OTHER NAME(S):   Woolsorter's disease, inhalation anthrax, cutaneous anthrax

Causative Organism: <u>Bacillus anthrasis</u>

Characteristics of Organism:
    Gram-positive bacillus
    Large - 4 to 8 micrometers by 1.5
        micrometers
    Aerobe
    Catalase - positive
    Non-motile
    Non-hemolytic
    Spore former - very resistant to drying
    Encapsulated - usually contains
      D- glutamic acid
    Virulence - Toxins

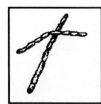

Endospore forming rods of <u>Bacillus anthrasis</u>

<u>Bacillus anthrasis</u> light area spores

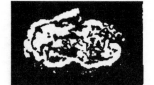

Colony of <u>B. anthrasis</u>

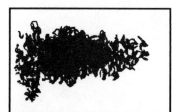

Colony of <u>Bacillus anthrasis</u>

Portal of Entry:
    Contact
    Inhalation
    Ingestion

Clinical Symptoms
    Multiple forms
       1. Cutaneous (malignant pustule)
           swollen, hemorrhage lesions
                 (non-pyogenic)
           Satellite vesicles develop
                 edema
           Develops eschar
           Spread to blood rare,

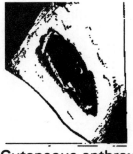

Cutaneous anthrax

               less than 5%
           Regional lymph adenitis and
             septicemia -
           poor prognosis

       2.   Pulmonary
           High fever
           Difficulty
              breathing

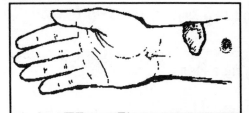

Cutaneous anthrax - skin lesion

           Pleurisy
           Pneumonic
             sepsis
           Clots pulmonary capillaries
           Lymphadenopathy
           Obstruction of airways
           Can lead to septicemia
                   meningitis
                   intestinal
           Toxins cause capillary thrombosis
           cardiovascular shock

       3.   Intestinal
           enteritis
           high mortality

Diagnosis:
    Cultural -   on blood agar
                    EYA (egg-yolk agar)
                     Curly hair-lock colonies

    Phase - Typing

Serology -   Ascoli Test

Treatment:
        Penicillin
        Tetracycline
        Erythromycin
        Chloramphenicol

Note: Onset of septicemia negates antibiotic effectiveness

Epidemiology:
        Animal vaccine can give anthrax to humans, problem for
        veterinarians

Other Bacilli causing diseases
        B. subtilis
            Endophthalmitis
            Right - side endocarditis
            Meningitis

        B. cereus
            Gastroenteritis
            Frequently, cooked improperly stored rice is the source

NAME OF DISEASE: Gas Gangrene
OTHER NAME(S):   Myonecrosis

Causative Organism: <u>Clostridium perfingens</u>
                        also Welch's Bacillus
                        <u>C. welchii</u>

        others <u>C</u> .<u>novyi</u>, <u>C</u>.<u>septicum</u>, <u>C</u>. <u>sporogens</u> and others

Characteristics of Organism:
        Gram-positive - bacillus (large)
        Strict anaerobe
        Spore former
        Encapsulated
        Non-motile
        Ferments -   Lactose
                      acid/gas
                      stormy fermentation
        Virulence - Toxins
           Alpha toxin - lecithinase
           20 myotoxins
           Hemolysin (theta toxin)
           Fibrinolysin
           Proteinase
           Neuraminidase
           Collagenase
           Hyaluronidase
           DNase

Portal of Entry: Wound

Clinical Symptoms:
        Incubation - 2 to 4 days
           Severe pain at wound site
           Edema
           Thick serosanguineous discharge
           Low grade fever
           Sweating
           Tachycardia

Lecithinase destroys capillary cell's
    membrane, affect permeability hemorrhage
Hemolytic anemia
Hypotension
Renal failure
Jaundice
Tissue turns black - fills with gas
Crepitation - tissue crackles on palpitation
Foul smell, dark exudate

Diagnosis:
    Clinical picture
    Microscopy - Diseased Tissue

Treatment:
    Antitoxin
    Surgical Debridement
    Penicillin, cefoxitin
    or amputation or
    Place patient in hyperbaric chamber
    at 3 atmospheres for 90 minutes
    2 or 3 times per day

Epidemiology
    Can occur at other times such in bowel when there are
    bowel obstructions or bowel surgery

    Pigbel, a disease (necrotizing enteritis) caused by Type C,
        C. perfringens, lack of protein in diet
        Abdominal pain/distention
        Vomiting
        Blood or black stools
        Areas of necrosis may result in bowel perforation
        Death or surgery a possibility
        Also cause cellulitis - inflammation of
                connective tissue
                erythema/edema

NAME OF DISEASE: Tetanus
OTHER NAME(S):   Lockjaw

Causative Organism: <u>Clostridia</u> <u>tetani</u>

Characteristics of Organism:
    Gram-positive bacillus
    Motile
    Spore - former - sensitive to sunlight
    Normal flora cow/horse manure
    Virulence - Toxins
      Tetanospasmin + plasmid yield
          neurotoxin
          exotoxin
      Neurotoxin - binds to
          ganglioside receptors of peripheral nerves
          travels via axons
          jump synapse to motor neuron
          block release of inhibiting neurotransmitter
          continuous contraction
    Organism itself not capable of producing damage and can
only infect necrotized cells

Portal of Entry:
    Break in skin

Clinical symptoms:
    Incubation - 2 days (severe) to 4 weeks (mild)
    Minimal inflammation
    Violent involuntary spasms can break bones
    Tonic spasm-resistant rigidity
    Risus sardonicus - continuous smile
    Trismus - painful spasms of jaw
    Tachycardia
    Hypertension
    Cardiovascular instability
    Chills/fever
    Leucocytosis
    Death could result respiratory impairment

In infant early sign is difficulty in suckling

Treatment:
>   Antitoxin   (TIGH) human tetanus immune globulin) or
>   heterologous tetanus antitoxin
>   Penicillin
>   Possible debridement
>   Muscle relaxants

Epidemiology:
>   Vaccine part of DPT

>   In third world countries can see tetanus neonatorum in infants - results of non-sterile severing of umbilical cord

NAME OF DISEASE: Hansen's Disease
OTHER NAME(S): Leprosy

Causative Organism: <u>Mycobacterium</u> <u>lepra</u>
also Hanesn's bacillus

Characteristics of Organism:
Acid-fast-bacillus
Filamentous
Obligate anaerobe
Non-motile
Non-spore forming
Difficult to impossible to culture in vitro
Generation Time - 12 days
(very slow grower)
Grows in cooler part of body-prefers
low temperature

Portal of Entry:
Inoculation
Inhalation
(organism shed in pus and with respiratory droplets)

Clinical Symptoms:
Incubation -
1 to 5 years- tuberculoid form
9 to 12 years- lepromatous form
Organism grown in peripheral nerves
and skin - two types
Organism phagocytized but not
destroyed

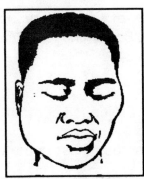

Ludwig's angina - jaw

1. Tuberculoid
Skin - large, erythematous
plaques
clearly defined border
become rough, hairless, hypopigmented
leave anesthetized scars
Nerves- peripheral nerves affected
small nerves - anesthesia
large trunk motor paralysis

Results -
- clawhand
- footdrop
- ocular complications

2. Lepromatous

Skin - lesions
small histiocyte infiltration around blood vessels
Maculas - indefinite border
hypo- or hyperpigmentation
Develop into plaques
- large, ill-defined, elevated flat called lepromas
- advanced state - cause facies leonina (Lionface)

Hepatosplenongaly
orchitis
loss of bone especially end of fingers and toes

Lepromatous Leprosy

Both forms of secondary forms called Borderline Tuberculoid, Borderline lepromatous

Predisposition:
- Environmental - Prolonged contact
- Genetic
- Sexual - Lepromatous most common in males

Complications:
- Erythema nodosum leprosum
- Lucio's phenomenon - punch out ulcers
- Secondary bacterial infections

Diagnosis:

Microscopic -   skin scrapings
                 Acid Fast Test
Serology -   Lepromin Skin Test
Clinical -   Fenther Test - numbness
                 also earlobes - for loss of heat -
                 cold sensitivity

Treatment:

Dapsones, a sulfone
    (dianimodiphemyl sulfane)
Rifampin
Clofazimine

Epidemiology:

15,000,000 cases would wide
over 2,500 cases in United States with 200-400
    new cases per year
United States cases localized Hawaii, Texas,
    Louisiana, Florida, California
1 of 200 exposed may get disease -
    not highly contagious
If individual has low resistance usually
    develops lepromatous
If individual has high resistance usually
    develops tuberculoid

249

NAME OF DISEASE: Psuedonomal infections

Causative Organism: <u>Pseudomonas</u> various species

Characteristics of Organism:
      Gram-negative - bacillus
      Oxidizes glucose (no fermentation)
      Grows in quaternary ammonium detergents
      Grows well at 42°C
      Grows at cold temperatures (refrigerator)
      Resistant to dyes
      Resistant to chlorine
      Produces a water-soluble blue-green pigment, pyocyanin -
          Fluoresces
      Polar flagella - motile
      Oxidase positive
      Catalase positive
      Virulence factors -
          mucoid capsule
          Enzymes - protease
                    amylase
                    pectinase
                    cellulase
        Hemolysin
        Endotoxin
        Exotoxins
      Sweet odor

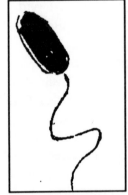

<u>Pseudomonas</u>
<u>aeroginosa</u>

      500 species

Portal of Entry: Dependent on disease
                  Wounds
                  Ingestion
                  Respiration
                  Contact

Predisposition: Burns
                    Skin wounds
                    Urinary catheters
                    Cancer chemotherapy
                    Cystic fibrosis
                    Elderly

Clinical Symptoms:
      Pseudonomal pyoderma - skin ulcers
                    punched out borders
                    blue-green pus
                    grape-like odor

      Classic ecthyma gangrenosum -
                    blisters with pink to violet halos
                    turn greenish-blue
                    to black

      Pseudomonal pneumonia -
                    blue-green sputum

      Otitis externa -   "Swimmers ear"

      Pseudomonal dermatitis - self-limiting rash
                    2 weeks
                    associated with pools and sauna

      Pseudonomal colitis - <u>Clostridia</u> <u>difficule</u>
                    watery diarrhea after use of antibiotics
                    abdominal pain
                    fibrin, mucous, WBC
                    in colon form
                    pseudomembrane
                    high mortality 25%

      Pseudomonal septicemia -
                    endotoxins in blood

Melioidosis -   <u>Pseudomonas</u> <u>pseudomallic</u>
                       Other names - Rangoon beggar's
                       disease, Whitmore's disease,
                       "Vietnamese time bomb"
          2 forms

                  1. Chronic - osteomyelitis
                                 respiratory
                                 radiologically   like
                                    tuberculosis
                  2. Acute -   pneumonia
                                bacteremia
                                high fever/chills
                                myalgia
                                hemoptysis
                                macuporurlent sputum
                                hepatosplenomegaly-
                                   jaundice
                                possible shock

Glanders -   <u>Pseudomonas</u> <u>mallei</u>
                       Reservoir horse

          Acute -   papule at site of initiation
                       bacteremia
                       fever
                       vomiting
                       generalized pain

          Chronic -   low grade fever
                       draining abscesses and lymph
                          nodes
                       lymphadenopathy
                       hepatosplenomegaly

Treatment - Sulfa drugs
Acute usually fatal
Mortality if chronic about 50%

Treatment:
- Carbenicillin*
- Ticarcillin*
- Gentamicin*
- Tetracycline*
- Silver sulfadiazine (Silvardene)
- Mafenide
- Topical colisthimelthate sodium
- Topical polymyxin B
- Debridement

* Multiple drug resistant organism

NAME OF DISEASE: Staphylococcal Skin Infections

Causative Organism: <u>Staphylococcus</u> various species

Characteristics of Organism:
    See Staphylococcal pneumonia

Virulence factors:
    Exotoxins - hemoplysims - 4 types
                  alpha toxins
                  beta toxins
                  gamma toxins
                  delta toxins
                  leucocidin

              Enterotoxins - 5 types

              Exfoliative Toxin
              Toxic Shock Syndrome Toxin I (TSST I)
    Survives in pus for months

Predispositions:
    Decreased resistance
    Burns/Ulcers
    Decreased blood flow to region
    Underlying skin disease

Clinical Symptoms:
    Furuncles -
            localized swellings
            soft-centers
            pyogenic-yellow
                 discharge

    Carbuncles -
            painful, red, indurated
            lesions form abscesses -
            large, spreads
            can lead to septicemia

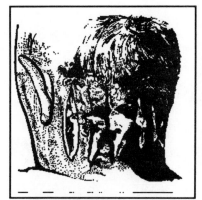

Carbuncle of
<u>Staphylococcus</u> aureus

Follicultits -
    infection around hair follicle
    pyogenic
    (pimples or pustules)
    on eyelash - called sty

Impetigo -
    superficial skin lesions
    macule to vesicle with pus

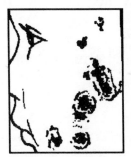

I m p e t i g o
contagiosum

Bone infection -
    osteomyelitis
    fever/chills
    pain in muscle
    spasms
    tender lumps
    necrosis of bone
    associated with traumatic injury

Scaled Skin Syndrome (SSS) -
    via toxin
    first lesion around mouth
      and nose
    develops as bright red
      area (within 48 hours)
    high fever
    skin peals off -
        palms and soles
    dry scale
    then rest of body
    can result in
        septicemia
        vomiting
        fever
        sunburn like rash
        shock

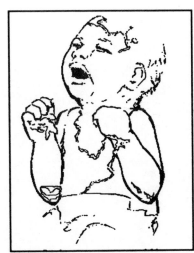

Scaled Skin Syndrome
(SSS)

Urinary tract infection - Staphylococcus saprophticus
    Common in sexually active women

Diagnosis:
>Coagulase Test
>Cultural -   Mannitol Salt
>Microscopic - Gram stain
>Antibiotic Sensitivity testing (some have penicillinase)

Treatment:
>Penicillin or drug after multiple sensitivity testing

NAME OF DISEASE: Erysipeloid
Causative Organism;   <u>Erysipelothrix</u> <u>insidiosa</u>
                      or <u>Erysipelothrix</u> <u>rhosiopathiae</u>

Characteristics of Organism:
       Gram-positive - bacillus
       Non-spore forming
       Non-motile
       Two forms -   single cell in short chains
                             long-branching filamentous chains

Portal of Entry:
       Break in skin
       source - contaminated food
       reservoir - Pig's tonsils

Clinical Symptoms:
       Limited to hands
       Swelling
       Inflamed dark red lesions
       Burning/itching

Complications:
       Septicemia
       Endocarditis

Diagnosis:
       Fermentation tests
       Mouse Protection Test

Treatment:
       Penicillin
       Erythromycin

OTHER BACTERIAL

DISEASES

Lyme's Disease
Human Bite Wounds
Acne Vulgaris
Tropical Phagedenic Ulcer

NAME OF DISEASE: Lyme's Disease

Causative Organism: <u>Borrelia</u> <u>burgdorferi</u>

Characteristics of Organism:
    Spirochete

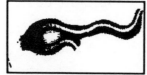

Borrelia
Gurgdorferi

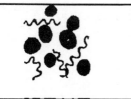

Borrelia
in blood

Portal of Entry:
    Break in skin
    Vector - hard ticks <u>Ixodes</u>
    Reservoir deer/mice - alternate
        (don't get symptoms)

Clinical Symptoms:
    Two stages
    1. Rash at site of bite
        forms bull's eye
            (erythema chronicum
                migrans)
            Fever
            Headache
            Stiff neck
            Dizziness
            Swollen lymph nodes
    2. Cardiac dysrthythmias
        Facial palsy
        Polyarthritis
        Takes 1 to 2 years to develop

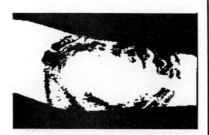

Lesion of Lyme's Disease
Bull's eye form

Complications:
      Encephalitis
      Myocarditis
      Alzheimer like symptoms, demyelination

Treatment:
      Penicillin
      Tetracycline
      Doxycline

Epidemiology:
      Can cross placenta
      Vaccine for dogs

NAME OF DISEASE: Cat Scratch Fever
OTHER NAME (S):   Maladie des giffes de chat

Causative Organism: CSD Bacillus

Characteristics of Organism:
    Gram-negative - Filamentous rods
    Up to 10 micrometers
    Difficult to culture
    Stain with silver impregnation techniques
    L-form during infection

Portal of Entry:
    Break in skin
    Reservoir - possibly cats

Clinical Symptoms:
    Incubation - 3 to 14 days
        Raised red nodule at site
        Swollen, tender lymph nodes
        Regional lymph adenopathy
        Last 3-4 months, may drain
        Fever
        Malaise
        Splenomegaly - rare
        Rash/erythema nodosum

Diagnosis:
    Skin test
    Contact with cat

Treatment:
    Symptomatic
    Surgical excision of nodes
    Possibly - Tetracycline

NAME OF DISEASE: Human bite wounds infections

Causative of Organism: <u>Ekinella</u> <u>corrodes</u>

Characteristics of Organism:
      Normal Flora
      Grow on agar + increased
            carbon dioxide

Portal of Entry:
      Breaks in skin
      via human bite

Clinical Symptoms:
      Cellulitis
      Osteomyelitis
      Bacteremia

Treatment:
      Penicillin

NAME OF DISEASE: Acne vulgaris

Causative Organism: <u>Propionibacterium vulgaris</u>

Characteristics of Organism:
    Forms free fatty acids
    causes inflammation

Clinical Symptoms:
    Non-inflammatory lesions - conedomes
        if open called - blackheads
        if closed called - white heads

    Severe acne -   cystic acne
                    inflamed cyst
                    severe scarring
                    ducts plugged

    If caused by staph called sycosis barbae and pustular acne vulgaris

NAME OF DISEASE: Tropical phagedenic ulcer

Causative Organism: <u>Bacillus fusiformis</u>
                           <u>Treponema vincentii</u>

Clinical Symptoms:
     Spreading, painful, sloughing ulcer
     raised border
     grey putrid exudate
     cup-shape center
     necrotizing
     Bones and tendons maybe come
visible

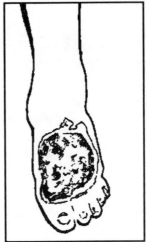

Tropical
phagedenic ulcer

Complications:
     Secondary bacterial infections
     Tibial osteomyelitis
     Squamous cell carcinoma

Treatment:
     Penicillin
     Sulfanilamide
     Tetracycline
     Metronidazole
     Reconstructive surgery

BACTERIAL DISEASE

OF THE

EYE

Hypopyon Keratitis
Acute maco-prurlent conjunctivitis
Septic Shock

NAME OF DISEASE: Hypopyon keratitis
OTHER NAME(S):   Chronic angular blephero-conjunctivitis

Causative Organism: <u>Moraxella</u> <u>lacunate</u>
    also Morax - Axenfeld Diplobacillus

Characteristics of Organism:
    Gram-negative - coccobacillus
    Motile-Flagellated
    Non-spore forming
    Oxidase positive
    Catalase positive
    Media with serum
    Unable to ferment glucose

Portal of Entry:
    Opportunist

Clinical Symptoms:
    Hypopyon keratitis - pus in anterior chamber of eye

    Chronic angular blepharoconjunctivitis -
        inflammation

Diagnosis:
    Cultural -   Loeffler's Media
    Microscopic -   Gram-stain
        Exhibit safety pin effect

Treatment:
    Penicillin

NAME OF DISEASE: Acute Maco-prurlent conjunctivitis
OTHER NAME(S):   Pink-eye, acute catarrhal
                      conjunctivitis, Brazil prurpric fever

Causative Organism: <u>Hemophilus</u> <u>aegyptii</u>
                      or Kock Weeks bacillus

Characteristics of Organism:
      See Haemophilic pneumonia

Portal of Entry:
      Direct contact
      Highly contagious

Clinical Symptoms:
      Pink inflammation of conjunctiva
      Copious discharge
            (dehydrates and crust while sleeping)
      Swollen eyes
      Photophobia

Diagnosis:
      See Haemophilic pneumonia - differentiated
      via Quellung test

Treatment:
      Penicillin

NAME OF DISEASE: Septic Shock

Causative agents:
Varied
Pseudomonas
Bacteroides Fragelis
Klebsiella
Proteus
Enterobacter
Serratia
Escherichia
Steptococcos
Staphylococcus
Actinomycoses

Portal of Entry:
Circulatory

Predisposition:
Immunodeficiency
Age
Trauma
Diabetes mellitus
Cirrhosis
Disseminated cancer

Clinical Symptoms:
Lymphangitis - inflamed lymph vessels
noted by red streaks
Fever - low grade
Nausea/vomiting
Thirst
Tachycardia
Tachypnea
Decreased peripheral blood circulation
Confusion
Extremities - cold and blue
Follow renal/cardiac failure
Coma
Death

Diagnosis:
    Clinical picture

Treatment:
    Restore fluids - circulatory system
    Antibodies

MYCOLOGICAL DISEASES

Superficial Mycosis
Subcutaneous Mycosis
Systemic Mycosis
Opportunistic Mycosis

CUTANEOUS MYCOSIS (MYCOSES: PL.)
ALSO REFERRED TO AS:

Superficial Mycosis
Dermatomycosis
Dermatophytosis

Tinea
Tinea nigra
Piedra
Favus
Tinea Versicolor

NAME OF DISEASE: Tinea (various)
OTHER NAME(S):   Ringworm

Causative agent(s):
hair
Genus <u>Trichophyton</u> also called <u>Anthroderma</u>
        (an ascomycetes)
Genus <u>Microsporum</u> also called <u>Nannizia</u>
        (an ascomycetes)
Genus <u>Epidermophyton</u>
        (a deutromycetes (Fungi imperfecti)

Characteristics of Organism:
     Dimorphic - yeast/mold form
     Saprophytic organisms of soil
     Utilize keratin - skin protein
        (have enzyme keratinase)
     Localized in superficial, dead, keratinized tissue
effects -   (hair, skin, nails)
     Each species has characteristic tissue(s) of infection
        <u>Trichophyton</u> - hair, skin, nails
        <u>Microsporum</u> - skin, nails
        <u>Epidermophyton</u> - hair, skin

Predisposition(s):
     moisture   perspiration
     warmth   sebum composition
     skin chemistry   exposure concentration
     genetic predisposition age

Portal of entry:
     Breaks in skin - Trauma
     Contact with spores - Direct
     Contact with spores - Indirect (fomites)
        clothing
        towels
        products of personal hygiene

Clinical symptoms:
      General: (one or more of the following)
            Inflamed itchy skin
            Circular scaly patches
            Peeling, cracking skin
            Ulcerative nodules
            Blister-like lesions, thin, fluid-filled
            Dry blisters
            Secondary reaction - hypersensitivity response
                    Dermatophytid Reaction
                       (Trichophytid Reaction)
                       Fungal products in non-infected site
                       Results - Eczema (Dermatitis)
                              Inflamed Vesicles (Itchy)

Specific Symptoms (Diseases)
    1. Tinea barbae
        "Barber's Itch"
        Most common organisms: <u>T. rubrum</u>
                                  <u>E. floccosum</u>
        Infection of bearded regions (men)
         Red, boggy (soggy) areas
         Annular scaly lesions
         erythema - red.
         Can be confused for pyogenic bacterial infection

    2.   Tinea Capitis
        "Ringworm of scalp"
        Most common organisms: <u>T. tonsurans</u>
                                 <u>M. audouinii</u>
                                 <u>M. canis</u>
         Juvenile type -
                Spotty patches
                Resolves at puberty (due to increase of fatty
                   acids)
                Inflammatory boggy masses

Severe inflammatory reaction called kerion, usually associated with <u>M. canis</u> that can be gotten from dogs or pets.

Ectothrix - Scaly, scattered lesions -shaft breaks - follicles with black centers - black-dot ringworm. *- outside of hair shaft*

Endothrix - infection within hair fiber *- Inside*

Adult form can lead to alopecia (baldness) *- condition*

3. **Tinea Corporis**

    Ringworm of Non-haired portions of body

    Most common organisms: <u>T. rubrum</u>
    <u>E. floccosum</u>

    circular patches
    central scaling
    red versicolor border

4. **Tinea Cruris**

    "Jock itch"

    "Dhobie Itch" *- severe form*

    Red, scaly, pruritic lesions

5. **Tinea Unguium**

    Onchymycosis *- under nail bed*

    Most common organisms: <u>T. rubrum</u>
    <u>T. mentagrophytes</u>

    Nails -   opaque, lusterless thickened, brittle
    pitted lesions
    white, patchy lesions
    discoloration

6. **Tinea manum**

    Ringworm of hands and palms

    Related to T. pedis

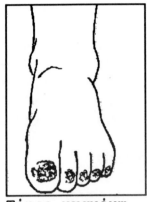

Tinea urguium

7. T. pedis
"Athlete's foot"
"Jungle rot"
Itchy, scaling
itchy, vesicles (blisters)
cracking of skin

usually adults

Course of Disease:
Spore land on skin or break in skin
Change to mold form
Hyphae penetrate surrounding tissue

＊ Types of Infection -
Anthropophilic - Human
to Human
Zoophilic - Animal to man, response to
treatment better, usually no reoccurrence

Diagnosis:

1. Skin Scrapings
Exposed to 10% warm NaOH or 20% warm KOH
Stains: Gram stain (very intense)
Periodic Acid Schiff (PAS) - magenta
Examine for micro- and macroconidia

Wood's LIGHT wavelength 365 greenish flares

Pyriform and
clavate
microconidia
of
Trichophyton

Trichophyton

microconidia -
pyriform, clavate
macroconidia -
smooth walled - *thinner*

Microsporum

microconidia - few
microconidia - rough
walled echinulate,
fusiform

8-15 compartments color = yellow/orangish

274

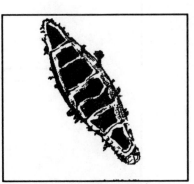

Echinulated, thick
walled spindled
macroconidia of
Microsporum

<u>Epidermophyton</u>   microconidia -
                          clavate
                  (club - oval - shaped)

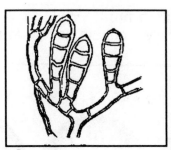

Clavate
macroconidia of
<u>Epidermophyton</u>

1-5 compartments
greenish/yellow

this
color under orange

2.   Nutritional studies

3.   Wood's light - ultraviolet light at 365 nm-
            Greenish Fluorescence - <u>T. Schoenlienii</u>
            <u>Microsporum</u>

4.   Culture -   Sabouraud's with chloramphenicol and
                  cylohexamide-colony appearance and
                  spores.
                  Dermatophyte Test Medium - white
                  fluffy colonies - turn red - positive test

Treatment:
   Topical Antifungals -
      Miconazole   Haloprogin   *Immidazle*
      Tolnaflate   Logamel
      Clotrimazole   Thiabendazine   *SOAP*
      Zinc Undecyclinate   Whitefield's Ointment   *high pH make*
      Potassium Permanganate   (Salicylic - Benzoic Acid)   *ANTi Fungal*

other -
Decrease humidity (Towel)
Alter ph
Ultraviolet light (365 nm.)
Griseofulvin - orally - only in severe infections - usually nail
     bed.

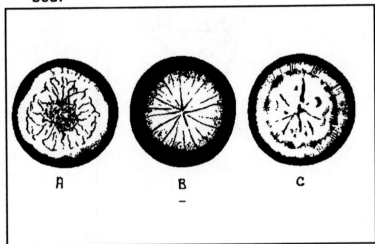

Colony of Dermatophytes

a. <u>Trichophyton</u>
b. <u>Microsporum</u>
c. <u>Epidermophyton</u>

NAME OF DISEASE: Tinea Nigra
OTHER NAME(S):   Tinea Palmaris

Black Ringworm

Causative Organism(s): <u>Cladosporium</u> <u>werneckii</u>
                      <u>Cladosporium</u> <u>mansonii</u>
                      Sexual phase - <u>Exophilia</u> <u>werneckii</u>

grows on outside

Clinical Symptoms:
    Flat, irregular, darkly discolored regions on palms of hand
    color darkest at periphery
    May resemble melanoma

Could Be misdosed

Diagnosis:
    On Sabouraud's - greenish-black colonies
    Skin Scrapings - Treated 20% NaOH/10%
                           KOH - warmed
                  Brown pigmented, branching, septated
                  hyphae
                  budding yeast cells

Treatment:
    Topical Ketolytic Solutions
        e.g. sulfur, salicylic acid, tincture of iodine

Epidemiology:
    Most common
        In Florida *, below JACKSONVILLE*
        95% cases teenagers
        of teenager cases - 75% female

NAME OF DISEASE: Piedra (Two Forms)
                               Black Piedra
                               White Piedra
OTHER NAME(S): Tinea Nodosum

Causative Organism(s):
         Black Piedra - Piedraia hortai
         White Piedra - Trichosporum beigelli
                            Trichosporum cutaneum

Clinical Symptoms:
     Black Piedra:
         Hard black nodules on hair shaft adhere tightly
     White Piedra:
         Soft, light-colored lesions on hair shaft easily lifted
             off

Diagnosis:
     Cultural - Sabouraud's Agar
         P. hortai - black to greenish-black colonies
                   colonies - wrinkled, glabrous
         T. beigelii - soft, cream-colored colonies
                   wrinkled
                   yeast-like

Treatment:
     Remove (shave) hair
     Apply: Solution of Mercuric Bichloride (1:2000) or
             ammoniated Mercury Ointment (3%)

NAME OF DISEASE: Favus (an endothrix)

Causative Organism: <u>Trichophyton</u> <u>schoenleini</u>
also called <u>Anthroderma</u> <u>schoenleini</u>

Clinical Symptoms:
Major Feature - Scutula
cup shaped crusts
yellowish
base of hair shaft
a mass of mycelial-epithelial debris

Complication:
Baldness

Treatment:
Topical agents: see Tinea

NAME OF DISEASE: Tinea Versicolor
OTHER NAME(S):   Pityriasis versicolor

Causative Organism(s):   <u>Malassia</u> <u>Furfur</u>*
                       <u>Pityrosporium</u> <u>orbiculares</u>*
        *Disagreement if different or the same organism:
part of normal skin flora

Predispositions:
    Excessive perspiration
    Corticosteroid Therapy
    Malnutrition
    Heredity
    High humidity

Clinical Symptoms:
    Lesions -   scaly, inflammatory
                   non-itching/itching
                   irregular, circumscribed
                   brownish-red
                    (area may be hyper- or de-pigmented)
                   fluoresces yellow under Wood's light
                   loss of pigment
                   residual - yellow to faun colored, grainy
                         patches

Diagnosis:
    Cultural -   Sabouraud's Agar with penicillin and
                    streptomycin
                 But organisms can also be cultured from
                    normal skin
                 Non - conclusive
    Microscopic - 10% warm KOH
                 Round budding cells
                 short unbranded hyphae
    Wood's Light - Golden - yellow fluorescence

Treatment:
    Weak ketolytic agents

SUBCUTANEOUS MYCOSIS (MYCOSES PL;)

Sporotrichosis
Chromoblastomycosis
Madura's Foot
Rhinosporidiosis

NAME OF DISEASE: Sporotrichosis
OTHER NAME (S):   Rose gardener's Syndrome (disease)

Causative Organism: <u>Sporothrix</u> <u>Schneckii</u>

Characteristics of Organism:
    Class - <u>Deutromycetes</u> (Fungi
        imperfecti)
    Cigar-shaped yeast cell (1-2 um by
        4-5 um) at 37°C or slightly
        less
    Found in mononuclear lymphocytes
    Dirty to white cottony mass on
        Sabouraud's at 25°C
    Flowered arrangement of conidia on
        conidiophore

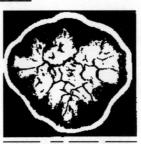

Colony of
<u>Sporothrix</u>
<u>schneckii</u>

Portal of Entry:
    Break in skin - puncture
                insect bites
                catfish strings
    (Organism associated with rotting
        wood, mulch, moss,
        sphagnum, etc.)
    Respiratory route - secondary portal

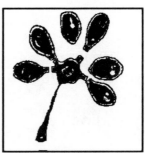

Condiospore of
<u>Sporothrix</u>
<u>schneckii</u>

Clinical Symptoms:
    Incubation - 1 week to 3 months
    average 3 weeks

    Three forms of the disease
        Lymphocutaneous sporotrichosis
        Extracutaneous sporotrichosis
        (Respiratory)
        Disseminated sporotrichosis

    Lymphocutaneous -
        Initially, small, moveable, firm nodule
        Nodule discolors to pink-purple

        Ulcerates, pus filled
        Necrotic
        Remains localized - (cutaneous sporotrichosis)
        Spreads along lymph channel
        Forms satellite nodules
        localized edema
Pulmonary (Respiratory)
        Productive cough
        lung cavities/nodules
        Hilar adenopathy
        Pleural effusion
        fibrosis
        Possibly a fungal ball

Disseminated
        Immunologically compromised patients
        Weight loss/anorexia
        bone lesions
        Complications - osteomyelitis, arthritis

Diagnosis:
    Cultural-   Sabouraud's Agar
                 25°C - creamy to white cottony mass
                 Pigment along periphery
                 Specimens from - pus, sputum, biopsy,
                    aspirations
                 Cystine Agar
                 37°C - yeast like colonies
                 BHI Agar
                 37° - pasty, grayish colonies

    Microscopic - Periodic acid schlif (PAS) or Methenamine
                   silver
                 Arrangement of conidia
                 Shaped and size of yeast cells

    Serology -   Fluorescent Antibody Test
                 Yeast cell agglutination Test
                 Exposure to - sporotrichum skin test

Treatment:

Cutaneous - Application of saturated Potassium Iodine for 1-2 months

Lymphocutaneous - Oral Potassium iodine from milk or O.J. - 4-6 weeks after recovery
Also ketoconazole, miconazole, fluconazole, itraconazole

Heat - palliative for pain
Organism heat sensitive - adjunct therapy

Extracutaneous - Amphotericin B
Surgical intervention - cavitary pulmonary lesions

Epidemiology:

Occupational risk - florist, gardeners, nursery workers
High Incidence - Mexico
In U.S. - Most common-Northeast

NAME OF DISEASE: Chromoblastomycosis
OTHER NAME(S): Chromomycosis, Verrucoses dermatitis

Causative Organism(s): <u>Phialophora</u>
<u>Cladosporium</u>
<u>Fonsecaea</u>

Characteristics of Organism:
General
Thick-walled, spherical bodies
6-12 microns
Produce melanin like pigments
Organism colors - olive-green, brown, black
Reservoir - soil

Portal of Entry: Break in skin

Clinical Symptoms:
Incubation - up to two or three years
Initially - small wart-like pustule, not painful
Becomes - raised, scaly, gray
Occasionally - Edema of hands and/or feet
Lymph drainage blocked
Minimal discomfort
Lesions can fuse to form - cauliflower-like granulomas

Complications: Neurotropic effects (rare)

Diagnosis:
Cultural -
Sabouraud's Agar
Slow, smoky/dark growth
Three types of conidiospores
Arotheca - oval spores on side of
Conidiophore - <u>Fonsecaea</u>
Spores at end of conidiophore-
<u>Cladosporium</u>
Philaspore - oval conidia on flask shaped
conidiophore - <u>Phialophora</u>

285

Skin Scrapings -   10% warm Potassium Hydroxide
                   Brown - hyphae
                   Thick walled Chlamydospore

Treatment:
    Sodium Iodine - intravenously
    Potassium Iodide - orally
    Sulfa/antibiotics to prevent secondary bacterial infections
    Surgical debridement
    Severe - amphotericin B and thiabendazole

Note: Can be confused with yaws

NAME OF DISEASE: Madura's Foot
OTHER NAMES(S):   Eumycetoma, if by Fungus
                            Mycetoma, if by fungus or bacteria
                            Actinomycetoma, if by <u>Actinomyces</u>

Causative Organism(s):
    Fungi: <u>Madurella</u>
                 <u>Monosporium</u>
                 <u>Petriellidium</u>
    Bacteria: <u>Actinomyces</u>
                 <u>Nocardia</u>

Portal of Entry: Break in skin (trauma)

Clinical Symptoms:
        Formation of Abscesses
        Edema/swelling
        Draining Fistulas - contain granules or microcolonies which
                are organisms enmeshed in a mucopolysaccharide
                protein matrix
        Steep-walled, punched out lesions
        Necrosis of small bones
        Deformation - formation of club foot
            (remains localized)

Diagnosis:
    Pus - dark grains
             hyaline/pigmented hyphae
             colored granules

Treatment:
        Varies by causative organism

Epidemiology:

        Most Common - Northern/Tropical Africa
                         Southern Asia
                         Tropical Americas

Lesions other than feet from vegetation or frequently burlap sacks carried by workers on shoulders.

Possible spread via sinus tracts to bone and muscle with loss of structure and function.

NAME OF DISEASE: Rhinosporidiosis

Causative Organism: <u>Rhinosporidium</u> <u>seeberi</u>

Characteristics of Organism:
      Globular sporangia - 10-30 micrometers
      Young, tropic form - 10-100 micrometers with central
         basophilic nucleus
      Spores - chitinous walls
         8-10 micrometers
         with 8-10 eosinophilic bodies

Portal of Entry: Unknown, possibly trauma

Clinical Symptoms:
      Can affect rectum, gentilia, larynx,
         conjunctiva and skin, but mostly
         nose

Nasal polyp of
Rhinosporidosi
Note: sporangia

     In nose -   Painless itching
                Mucoid discharge
                Lesions develop on
                   mucosa
                Become   hyperplastic,
                   polyploidic mass
                Soft, nodular, reddish

masses

                Bleeding
                May distract breathing or protrude from pores

     On skin -   Thick warty lesion

     On Conjunctiva -
                tearing
                discharge
                redness
                photophobia

Diagnosis:
    Microscopic - Biopsy
                      Round, thick-walled sporangia in white granulated tissue with plasma cells, lymphocytes, focal areas of histiocytes and neutrophils

Treatment:
    Surgery
    Cauterization

Epidemiology:
    Source - Possibly fish, insects or fresh water
             Associated with scuba diving
             Young adults - 90% male
        Most Common in India and Sri Lanka

Systemic Mycosis (Mycoses, pl.)

ALSO REFERRED TO AS:
DEEP - SEATED MYCOSIS

Cryptococcosis
Histoplasmosis
Coccidioidomycosis
Paracocidioidomycosis
Blastomycosis
Geotrichosis
Mucormycosis
Cladosporiosis
Aspergillosis
Mycotoxicosis

NAME OF DISEASE: Cryptococcosis
OTHER NAME(S):   Torulosis, European blastomycosis
                  Specific Form = Torulan meningitis

Causative Organism: Cryptococcus neoformans
                         previous name - Torula neoformans
                         sexual form - Filobasidiella neoformans

Characteristics of Organism:
        A basidiomycetes
        Four serotypes
        Thick capsule prevents
            phagocytosis, virulent
        Temperature sensitive - grows at
            37°C - no growth at 41°C
        At 37°C-budding yeast cells
        Found in soil-high concentration
            pigeon droppings, uses creatinine
        Bird-reservoir, unaffected due to
            body temperature
        Carbohydrates - non - Fermentative
        Hydrolyzes starch
        Assimilates inositol
        Urease positive

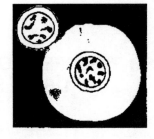

The large capsule of Cryptococcus neoformans

Portal of Entry:
        Respiratory system - inhalation of
        aerosolic bird feces

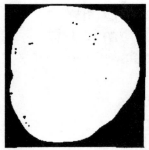

Moist, slimy, mucoid (cream-colored) yeast-like growth of Cryptococcus

Clinical Symptoms:
        Pulmonary cryptococcosis -
            asymptomatic or Flu-like or
            rare - Tuberculosis-like
        Possibly fungal ball called
            cryptococcoma -
            circumscribed nodule, necrotic center, heals with no
            calcification

Cryptoccocal meningitis -

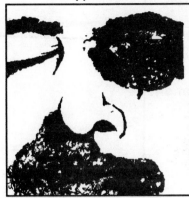

Cryptococcosis

severe frontal temporal
　　headache
low grade fever
stiff neck
diplopia
dizziness
Ataxia/paralysis
vomiting
memory loss
convulsions
eventually-untreated
　　coma
death - cerebral edema or
　　hydrocephalus
(Usually in immunologically comprised patients)
Skin lesions
Bone - painful osseous lesions
Brain - Abscesses
Tumor - like lesions

Complications:
　　optic nerve atrophy
　　permanent ataxia
　　deafness
　　paralysis
　　chronic brain/memory problems

Diagnosis:
　　　　Microscopic - Biopsy and fluids

　　　　Stains -　　India ink
　　　　　　　　　Nigrosin
　　　　　　　　　Mucicarmine - capsule bright red
　　　　　　　　　Alcian blue
　　　　　　　　　Capsule appears as a halo
　　　　　　　　　Two or three times thickness of cell

Cultural -   Sabouraud's Agar
                  with phenol, produces melanin
                  without - white, glistening mucoid
                      colonies

Serology -   Latex Cryptococcal Agglutination
                  Quelling Reaction

Spinal Tap -   Increased opening pressure
                  Increased monocytes
                  Elevated protein
                  Decreased glucose
                  Decreased chloride

Treatment:
  Pulmonary form - unnecessary
          Meningitis -   Amphotericin B
                            Intrathecal
                            Three - six months
                                 or
                            Amphotericin B
                            Flucytosine

NAME OF DISEASE: Histroplasmosis
OTHER NAMES(S):   Summer flu, Darling's Disease, Ohio Valley
                   Disease, Spelunkonosis, Central Mississippi
                   Valley   Disease,   Retieuloenththeliosis,
                   Appalicachian Mountain Disease (7)

Causative Organism: Histoplasma capsulation
                       also called Ajellomyces capsulatum

Characteristics of Organism:
    Dimorphic - 25°C -   Mold form
                  Tuberculated
                     microconidia
              called aleuriospores
               37°C - Yeast form
              grows in macrophages,
                 blood cells
              two - four micrometers
    Grows in guano - rich soil - high
              sodium content
    In soil - temperature, humidity - sensitive

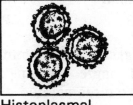

Histoplasmal
tuberrulated
macroconidia

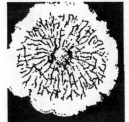

Yeast stage
colony of
Histoplasma

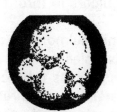

Wooly growth
on agar of room
temperature of
Histoplasma
capsulation

Portal of Entry:
    Respiratory -   inhalation of
                    spores/hyphae
    Reservoirs -   Birds not susceptible
                    Bats - susceptible

same body temp as human

This region

dry fecal material

295

Clinical Symptoms:
    Incubation period three - twenty days
    Three types:

1. Primary Acute histoplasmosis
    Resembles a mild respiratory infection or flu

fever	myalgia
headache	anorexia
cough	pleurisy

2. Progressive disseminated histoplasmosis also called acute disseminated histoplasmosis or chronic disseminated disease.
    Affects Reticuloendothelial System

Lymphadenopathy	Dysphagia
hepatosplenomegaly	leucopenia
anorexia	weakness
ulcers in throat	fever

3. Chronic pulmonary (cavitary) histoplasmosis
    Resembles tuberculosis
    Persist two - three months
    Cough, blood - tinged sputum
    dyspnea
    hemoptysis
    elevated temperature, night sweats
    hoarseness
    pleurisy

Histoplasmoma - two - three cm., central area of necrosis within fibrocytic capsule, calcifies.

Complications: Endocarditis
                  Meningitis
                  Necrosis of liver, spleen, bone marrow, heart

Diagnosis

Cultural - Blood Agar slants - 37∘C
Yeast like colonies, netted appearance
Slow growing - eight - twelve weeks
Sabouraud's Agar - 25∘C
White cotton colony, changes to buff color,
silky, aerial hyphae

Microscopic - Tissue sections - stained
Gram
Wright
Geimsa
Methenamine silver (Gomori's)

Serology - Complemenation Fixation Test
Immunodiffusion

Sensitivity Test - Histoplasmin skin test delayed
hypersensitivity test using crude
extract of mycelium grown on artificial
media (cross - reacts with Blastomycin
and Coccidioidin Skin tests)

Treatment:

Amphotericin B - (eight to ten weeks)
Ketoconazole
(Limits progression - no restoration of function)
Surgical removal nodules, histoplasmomas
External oxygen

Epidemiology:
H. dubuisii - African Form
cutaneous ulcers/nodules
Lymphadenopathy
Lesions of long bones and skull
Visceral lesions
No lung involvement

297

Histoplasmosis -   Mostly affects males over 50
                     children - primary, acute

In some regions Mississippi/Ohio Valley 95% of adults test
positive for exposure

As many as 40,000,000 maybe exposed per year resulting
     in 1,500 - 2,000 hospitalizations per year and leading to
     25 to 125 deaths per year.

Progressive disseminated disease - 70% fatal

Chronic pulmonary without treatment - 50% fatal

NAME OF DISEASE: Coccidioidomycosis
OTHER NAME(S):   California Disease, Desert Fever, Valley
                   Fever, San Joaquin Valley Fever, Desert
                   rheumatism (5)

Causative Organism: <u>Coccidioides</u> <u>immitis</u>

Characteristics of Organism:
    Dimorphic
    Forms -   Arthrospore in
                 mold form
                 characteristic
                 barrel - shape
                 with hyphae
                 section in
                 between

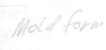
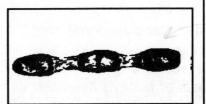

Coccidioidal arthrospore

    Spherule -   Capsules 20 - 60 micrometers containing
                 large number of endospores
    Prefers -   high carbon
                 high salt
                 semi-arid conditions
    Resistant - desiccation
                 temperature
                 loss of nutrients

Portal of Entry:
    Inhalation of spores

Clinical Symptoms:
    1. Incubation ten - sixteen days
       Primary acute
       Coccidioidomycosis
           Fever
           Cough
           General malaise
           Pleurisy
           Resembles Flu
       Resolves - three weeks - three months
           Later - Allergic Reactions - skin
                    (may or may not occur)

Coccidicidomycosis
nodular skin lesion

299

Erythema multiform, inflamed vesicles hemorrhage

hard   Erythema nodosum-subcutaneous
nodule - painful   *bone damage*
Also -   wart-like lesions - hypal
tunneling
arthralgia ("bumps")

2. Disseminated Coccidioidomycosis
Fever
Abscesses throughout body
Necrosis of bone, spleen and liver
Bone pain
Pulmonary cavitation with hemoptysis
Fungoma in lung

Complications:
Meningitis

Diagnosis:
Cultural -   Sabouraud's with chloramphenicol and
cycloheximide - 25°C
moist, white to brown colony
branching hyphae
flat, membranous
cottony, wooly aerial hyphae
forms arthrospore
(Caution: highly infectious - respiratory
precautions)
Converse media - 5% CO_2 - 37%
Growth of spherule
Sabouraud's - 30°C
Lactophenol cotton blue stain
Spores demonstrated

Serology -   Immunodiffusion
Tube precipitation
Complement - fixation
(Titre correlates to severity)

Hematology -   Increased lymphocytes
Increased eosinophils
Increased RBC Sedimentation

Sensitivity -   Skin test - Different extracts
Coccidioidin skin test
Spherulin skin test

Treatment:
Amphotericin B
Ketoconazole
Surgery if pulmonary involvement
Intrathecal if meningitis

Epidemiology:
Vaccine -   Levine's
Not available
Formalin treated spherule

Common among migrant workers

Predisposition -
Dark skin races
males - older
females third trimester of pregnancy
age extremes

Highest incidence -
Phoenix, Arizona
Tucson, Arizona
Kern Co, California

About 100,000 cases per year
50 - 100 deaths per year

NAME OF DISEASE: Paraccidioidomycosis
OTHER NAME(S):   South American Blastomycosis,
                   Paraciccidioidal Granuloma, Lutz-Splendor -
                   Almeida's Disease (3)

Causative Organism: Paracoccidioides braziliensis
                        also called Blastomyces brazilienis

Characteristics of Organism:
        Large, round thick walled yeast cells
        Multiple budding - buds remain attached
        Form pilot wheel arrangement
        Slow growing
        Characteristics vary
        Spore variable -   conidia
                            chlamydospore
                            arthrocondia
        Reservoir - Possibly soil

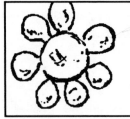
Paracoccidiodas

blastospores

2nd exposure

Portal of Entry:
        Inhalation - First infection usually inapparent
                      Reoccurrence due to possibly
                            Immunity
                            Diet or lack of
                            Age
                            Virulence of strain

Clinical Symptoms:

    1.   Muco-cutaneous Paracoccidioidomycosis
              papular vesicles that ulcerate particularly on
              mucosa of mouth, nose, rectal region
              Can spread via lymph
         lymphadenopathy - in mesteric lymph nodes could be
              confused for Hodgkin's disease
         Juvenile type - lymphadenopathy in lungs then to
              RES - could be fatal

2.   Benign Pulmonary Paracoccidioidomycosis
         Asymptomatic
         Identification via - skin test
         Residual calcification

3.   Progressive Pulmonary Paracoccidioidomycosis
         Resembles cavitary T.B.

Diagnosis
    Cultural -   Blood Agar or Beef Infusion Glucose
                      Agar at 37°C
                      Smooth waxy yeast-like colonies
                      Sabouraud's with or without antibiotics
                        at 25°
                      Short white aerial hyphae mycelium
                      changes to light brown chlamydospore

    Microscopic - From biopsy tissue, scrapings, aspirates
                      yeast - six - thirty micrometers
                           many smooth buds

    Serology -   Immunodiffusion
                      Complement fixation

Treatment
    Amphotericin B
    Ketoconazole
    Either combined with sulfa drugs
    Administration - 2⁺ years

NAME OF DISEASE: Blastomycosis
OTHER NAME(S): North American Blastomycosis, Gilchrist Disease, Chicago Disease

Causative Organism: <u>Blastomyces</u> <u>dermatitis</u>
also called <u>Ajellomyces</u> <u>dermatitis</u>

Characteristics of Organism:
<u>Ascomycetes</u>
Dimorphic
When budding forms a Figure "8" (yeast form)
Reservoir soil, mostly central
United States
Cells large, round refractile
5-15 micrometers
multiseptated
Also affect dogs, but not
animal reservoir

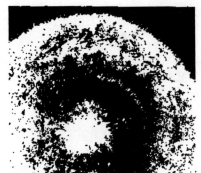
Mold form - giant colony
<u>Blastomyces</u>

Portal of Entry:
Inhalation dust, possibly pigeon droppings
Disease starts usually in mouth

Clinical Symptoms:
1. Cutaneous Blastomycosis

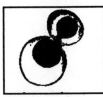
Budding in
<u>Blastomyces</u>
<u>dermatidis</u>

Raised wart-like blisters, small, painless become u l c e r a t i v e granulomas
Advancing borders
Discolored, crusty, lesions

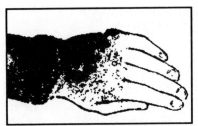
Blastomycosis

2. Subcutaneous Blastomycosis
Marked regional inflammation
necrosis, marked pyogenesis

304

3.   Pulmonary Blastomycosis
     Persistent cough - dry, hacking or productive,
         hemoptysis
     Pleurisy
     Fever and shaking chills
     Early stage radiography - T.B. or histoplasmosis
     Later stage radiography - crab-claw dark shadows

4.   Genitals/dissemination
     Painful swelling of testis
     Perianal pain
     Pyuria
     Hematuria

Complications: Meningitis
                 Addison Disease
                 Arthritis
                 Osteomyelitis

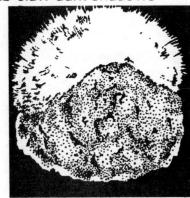

Yeast phase -
<u>Blastomyces</u>

Diagnosis:
   Cultural -   Blood Agar or
                     Brain Heart Infusion at 37°C
                     Soft, waxy, wrinkled colonies
                     Sabouraud's Agar - 25°C
                     White to light brown filamentous colony
                     Hyphae with aleuriospore on sides
                     Yeast extract agar with ethylene oxide
                     Sterilized bone meal-
                     Ascus visible containing light tan
                         uninucleated ascospore

   Microscopic -   Potassium hydroxide treated pus, sputum,
                         etc.
                     Oval, granular, refractile yeasts with
                         unipolar buds

Serology -   Complement-Fixation
              Immunodiffusion - better for two antigens
                  of <u>Blastomyces</u>

Skin Test -   Blastomycin Skin Test
              crude extract of mycelium

Treatment:
    Amphotericin B
    Hydroxystilbamidine isethionate
        (For cutaneous Form, less toxic)

Epidemiology:
    Associated with
            Age - middle
            Race - black
            Sex - male
            Housing - poor
            Occupation - dust, wood
            Nutrition - poor

NAME OF DISEASE: Geotrichosis

Causative Organism: <u>Geotrichum</u> <u>candidum</u>

Characteristics of Organism:
    Thick-walled, ovid yeast -
        1-15 micrometers
    Rectangular arthrospore in
        sputum
    Commensal in mouth,
        gastrointestinal and
        genito-urinary tract

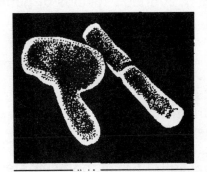

<u>Geotrichum</u> <u>candidum</u>

Portal of Entry:
    Respiratory

Clinical Symptoms:
    Respiratory - chronic bronchitis
              persistent cough
              Mucous - white, thick
                      grey flecks
                      blood-streaked
              fine to medium rales
              diffuse peribronchial thickening

Complications:
    Oral Geotrichosis - resembles thrush
    Otomycosis - puncture of eardrum

Diagnosis:
    Cultural -   Sabouraud's Agar - 25° or 37°C
                  Fast growth fungus
                  Membranous, mealy, flat, white, colony

Treatment:
    Potassium iodine - oral
    Sodium iodine - IV
    Aerosolized Nystatin

grows as mold not yeast

NAME OF DISEASE: Mucormycosis
OTHER NAME(S):   Phycomycocis, Zygomycosis

Causative Organism(s): Various species of genera
                        Mucor
                        Rhizopus   } zygomycetes
                        Absidia
                        Mortierella

Characteristics of Organism(s):
        Phycomycetes (zygomycetes)

        Hyphae in mycelium - broad, non-septated cyanotic
                10-30 micrometers in width
                Poorly stained with PAS
                highly-branching into tissues
                particularly vessels

Predisposition:
        Acidosis (Ketoacidosis) Diabetics
        Impaired phagocytosis
        Corticosteroid therapy
        Viremia
        Burn patient
        Malnutrition
        Leukemia
        Multiple myeloma
        long term, broad-spectrum antibiotics

Portal of Entry:
        Possibly Respiratory
        Possibly Mucous membrane

Clinical Symptoms:
        1. Neural Mucormycosis or Rhinocerbral Mucormycosis
                Meningoencephalitis
                Exopthalmia
                Interorbital cellulitis

Edema of face
Necrosis, hemorrhagic lesions on face
Fatal, swiftly

2. Pulmonary Mucormycosis
   Severe chest pain
   Pleurisy
   Bloody sputum
   Areas of consolidation, view or x-rays
   Fatal in 1-4 weeks
3. Circulatory
   Invasion of vessels by hyphae
   Thromboses, infarction, neuroses

Other forms cause by different organisms

Subcutaneous

Causative Organism: <u>Basidiobolus hystosporus</u>

Characteristics of Organism:
    Dimorphic
    Hyphae - non septated, thin-walled
              collapse

Clinical Symptoms:
    Enlarging, hard, inflammatory mass on shoulder, buttocks,
        thigh, trunk
    Well-defined edge lifts off easily

Treatment:
    Potassium Iodine

Nasofacial -
    Causative Organism -   <u>Entomophthora coronata</u>
    Clinical symptoms: Like subcutaneous, but on face
                            Disfiguring

Diagnosis:
    Microscopic - Tissue Section
                  Hematoxylin - Eosin
                  Observe - large, broad, non-separated
                  hyphae.

Treatment: Amphotericin B   (But most cases - 90% fatal)

310

NAME OF DISEASE: Cladosporiosis

Causative Organism: <u>Cladosporium</u> <u>bantianum</u>

Characteristics of Organism:
     Branching of separated, brown hyphae
     Hyphae cells - dumb-bell shaped

Portal of Entry:
     Respiratory

Clinical Symptoms:
     Neural -   Chronic Meningitis
               Headache
               Drowsiness
               Hemipeglia
               Brain Abscesses

Diagnosis:

     Cultural -   Sabourand's Agar - 25°C
                Olive gray to olive-brown
                Colony velvety surface
                Slow growing

     Microscopic - Tissue sections
                Hematoxylin - eosin
                Characteristic hyphae

Treatment:
     Non - Specific

Epidemiology:

Diagnosis frequently discovered at autopsy or after removal of abbess.

NAME OF DISEASE: Aspergillosis
OTHER NAME(S): Malx Worker's Disease

Causative Organism: <u>Aspergillus</u> <u>fumigatus</u>
<u>Aspergillus</u> <u>flavus-orgzae</u>
<u>Aspergillus</u> <u>niger</u>

Characteristics of Organism:
Mycelial - Hyphae growth only
Gray - green molds
Frequently associated with decaying food, damp hay, compost, moldy cereal grain
Risk to farmers, furriers, grainery workers, nursery employees

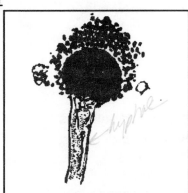

Aspergillan conidiospore

Predisposition:
Cancer - particularly leukemia, lymphoma, Hodgkin's
Corticosteroid therapy by macrophage suppression and neutropenia - Contraindicated during most forms of disease
Antibiotics - prolonged use
Irradiation and Immunosuppressive drugs
Alcoholism
Other cavitary respiratory illness

Portal of Entry:
Respiratory
Trauma, in a few instances, like eye

Clinical Symptoms:
1. Respiratory aspergillosis or aspergilloma
large ball of hyphae - invasive
Asymptomatic or resembles TB
productive cough
wheezing
blood - tinged sputum
fever/chills

       severe inflammation
       capillary breakdown
       hemoptysis
       night sweets
       X-ray - similar to neoplasm
       Mostly - <u>A</u>. <u>niger</u>
       Grows in warm, moist, well - aerated, protein rich environment, i.e. lung
       Hyphae - parallel or radial arrangement

2. Acute Aspergillosis-
       Usually <u>A</u>. <u>Fumigatus</u>
       Hyphae radial arrangement
       Necrosis of lung tissue
       Invasion of capillaries - thrombi
          (A humoral immune response)

3. Primary, Allergic Bronchopulmonary Aspergillosis
       Raised levels of IgE
       Eosinophilia
       Asthma
       Bronchial Constriction
       Productive cough
       Fever
       Prostration
       Dyspnea
       Pleurisy

4. Aspergillosis endopthalmitis (Keratomycosis)
       clouded vision
       pain
       reddened conjunctiva
       Infects anterior/posterior chambers producing portent exudate

5. Disseminated aspergillosis
       Cardiac - Thrombosis, infarcts
       CNS - Stroke, pyogenic meningitis
       Urinary tract obstruction

Skin - Thick nodular granulomas
        (Resembles Hansen's Disease)
Otomycosis - itching, swelling, sharp pain ear drum may rupture

Diagnosis:
    Cultural -   Sabouraud's
                        White cotton colony, becomes velvety
                        Spores create green powdery appearance

    Microscopic -   Tissue with stains
                            Periodic acid schiff
                            Gram's
                            Hematoxylin - Eosin

Treatment:
    Cutaneous -   Iodine compound
                        Nystatin
    Systemic -   Amphotericin B
                        Flucytosine
    Surgical -   Removal of Aspergilloma

NAME OF DISEASE: Mycotoxicosis

Causative Organism: Aspergillus favus

Characteristics of Organism:
      Hyphae/Mycelia growth form only
      Effect mediate via an endotoxin called aflatoxin - highly
            saturated molecule with coumarin nucleus
      Associated with moldy grains, peanuts and other
            underground crops
      Possibly also associated with some cheeses

Portal of Entry: Oral

Clinical Symptoms:

      Animals poisoned - meat contaminated diary products
            contaminated
      Humans - rarely have symptoms

Epidemiology:
      Suspected liver carcinogen based on studies in
            Uganda - diet based on peanut and people exhibit
            high level of liver tumors (up to 50%)
      FDA limit aflatoxin levels in peanut butter by regulation

OPPORTUNISTIC INFECTIONS

Candidal Infections

Candidiasis

NAME OF DISEASE: Candidiasis
OTHER NAME(S):   Moniliasis, Vaginitis, Vaginal Thrush,
                     Vulvovaginitis, Candidiasis (5)

Causative Organism: Candida albicans
                     used to be called Monilia albicans
                     Also other species - C. parapsisosis
                                          C. guillermondii

Characteristics of Organism:
    Dimorphic - yeast and hyphae -
        during tissue invasion
    Part of normal flora
    Buds elongate - remain attached
        called pseudohyphae

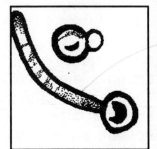

Candidal germ
term formation

Predisposition:
    Increased glucose as in diabetic
    Immunosuppressive drugs/radiation
    Aging
    Irritation of dentures
    Malnutrition
    Antibiotics and change in normal flora
    Changes cervical/vaginal mucosa
    Increased steroids

Portal of Entry - Contact
    One of the predisposition

Clinical Symptoms:
    Vaginitis -   Pruritus/itching
              White cheese discharge
              Burning internal pain on urination

    Skin -   Scaly, erthymatic rash, papular
              May be covered, exudate
              Below breasts, between fingers and toes
              Umbilicus, axillae
              Called Intertriginous candidiasis
              Cause - poor hygiene

bright white

pseudohyphae

yeast odor

Paronchyia - (Onchyia)
      Red, swollen nailbed
         (darkened)
      Possibly discharge -
         yellow
      Destruction of
         nail/nailbed
      hardening, browning,
         distortion

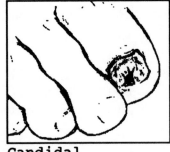

Candidal
orychomycosis

Thrush - (Black Hairy Tongue)
      Soft, crumbly milk like curds
      Cream colored/bluish-white patches
      Tongue and mouth scraped to expose bloody
      engorgement
      Possible gastroenteritis and diarrhea if affects
      G.I. tract

Chelitis - Scattered infective foci on lips

Stomatitis - Pursed lips
      grooves at corner of mouth

Systemic - Chills/high spiking fever
      Prostration
      Rash
      Hypotension

Bronchopulmonary - hemoptysis
      cough
      resembles miliary T.B.

Renal - Flank pain
      dysuria
      yeast odor to urine
      hematuria

Alimentary - diarrhea

Chronic Mucocutaneous -
  All surface tissue, dark, granulantous patches
  verrucous/warty, horn like lesions
  Immunodeficiency
  Addison Disease
  Hypoparathyroidism

Cutaneous - Factors; moisture,
  friction, warmth
  Occupational hazard

Candidemia -

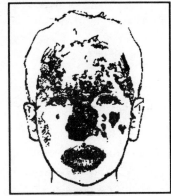

  Candida in blood
  Due to - Indwelling
    catheter
    Surgery
    Trauma

Mucocutaneous
candidiasis

Diagnosis:
 Cultural - Sabouraud's with antibiotics at 37°C
  Smooth, medium-sized (1-2mm) pasty colony,
  cream-colored
  yeast odor
  Levine-Eosin Methylene Blue Agar at 37°C
  Filamentous colony
  Cornmeal Agar - 37°C
  Chlamydospores visible

 Microscopic -
  Scrapings - treated warm alkali
  Strongly gram positive
  Pseudohyphae pinched at point of attachment

 Serology - Agglutination Test
  Immunodiffusion Test
  Indirect Immundofluoresscent Test
  Rapid yeast Identification System
  (12 tests - most reliable)

Chlorine does not kill protozoans.

PROTOZOAL DISEASES

4 Groups

Sarcodinian Diseases — *flesh eat*
Ciliophoran Diseases — *cilia*
Mastigophoran Diseases — *Flageli*
Sporozoan Diseases — *No Locomotion*

SARCODINIAN DISEASES

Amebiasis
Primary Amebic Meningoencephalitis
Acanthamebic Diseases

NAME OF DISEASE: Amebiasis
OTHER NAME(S):   Amebic dysentery, gastroenteritis
                         (general)

Causative Organism: *tissue*
    Entameba histolytica

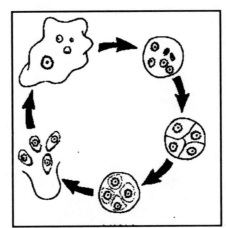

Life cycle Entameba
histolytica

- LARGE
numerous
pseudopods

Characteristics of Organism:
    Two stages

        Trophozoite stage
        (feeding form)
            8-60
                micrometers
            Extensive
                ectoplasmic
                pseudopodia
            Nucleus only visible with staining
            Ingests bacteria in colon and RBC's (visible
            within organism)
            Found in cecal area and ascending colon
            Not able to survive in outside environment
    Encysting
            Reorganization nuclear material
            Rounding of organism
            Reduction in size
            Becomes sluggish

        Cyst stage
            5-20 micrometers/spherical
            1-4 nuclei visible - each will become new
                trophozoite
            Cysts passes in feces
            Form of transmission
            Viable if kept moist
            Resistant to acid

322

Sensitive to desiccation, sunlight, and heat
Survive up to month in cool; moist
environment

Portal of Entry: Fecal - oral route
Anal intercourse
Contaminated colonic apparatus

Clinical Symptoms:
Acute amebiasis (amebic colitis)   — Colon
High fever - about 104°-105°F/chills
Abdominal cramping/tenesmus/flatulence
Profuse bloody diarrhea/mucous
Malodorous stools
Abdominal tenderness - due to ulcers
Ulcers -   non-inflammatory
flask-shape or tear drop
tissue invasion via lysis
grey-necrotic areas
sharp line between ulcer and
functional mucosa
late stages - presence of
neutrophils, lymphocytes,
histiocytes, eosinophils,
and plasma cells
severe case - anemia/emaciation

Chronic Amebiasis
Intermittent diarrhea - 1-4 weeks
Recurring
4-18 movements per day
Mild fever
Abdominal tenderness
Hepatomegaly

Ameboma/Amebic granuloma
Masses form
Can cause napkin-ring contraction or blockage
Mistaken for cancer, diagnosis via surgery
Bloody/mucous stools

Amebic hepatitis
>   Perforate bowel
>   Parasitemia
>   To liver, forms abscesses
>   Low grade fever
>   Leucocytosis
>   Liver enzymes - elevated
>   Serum protein - depressed
>   Tenderness
>   Referred pain - right scapula
>   Only parenchymal cells affected, not connective
>   tissue
>   Liquefaction of liver to creamy chocolate color
>   Eventually only lace-like connective tissue left

Cutaneous
>   Cauliflower-like lesions on skin

Penetration of diaphragm
>   Can result in -   pulmonary amebiasis
>   pericardial effusion
>   amebic pericarditis
>   cardiac failure

Diagnosis:
>   Microscopic -   Dysenteric material - dual preparations
>   Various stains and salt solutions
>   High and low power observation
>   Semi-formed stools - cysts
>   Dual preparation
>   D"Antoni's stain-internal structure
>   Salt solution - refractive cyst wall
>   Other stains - Iron hematoxylin
>
>   Serology -   Indirect hemagglutination (liver)
>   Commercial ELISA Kit
>
>   Sigmoidoscopy

Treatment:
> Metronidazole (Flagy)
> Emetine HCL (dihydroemetine) — *controlled in hospital*
> Chloroquine diphosphate (liver) (Aralen) — *Brand name*
> Paromomycin combined with others
> Iodoquinol (diiodohydroxyquin) - for carriers

Epidemiology:
> Human only reservoir
> Amebas not destroyed by chlorination, removed by filters
>> if functioning properly
> Disease endemic in United States - 5-10% population
>> affected
> World wide more than 100,000 deaths per year

TAKen for weeks

NAME OF DISEASE: Primary Amebic Meningoencephalitis
OTHER NAME(S):   PAM

Causative Organism: Naegleri Fowleri
                        also Naegleri gruberi

Characteristics of Organism:
        Flask shaped
        Single broad pseudopod
        Prominent feeding structure - amebostome
        Can be flagellated outside human
        Cyst and trophozoite form
        Exists in brackish water
        Resistant - freezing, chlorination

Portal of Entry: Mucus membranes of nose

Clinical Symptoms:
        Nasal congestion
        Headache
        Nausea/vomiting
        Fever
        Loss of sense of smell/taste
        Rigidity of neck
        Delirium
        Fulminating
                meningoencephalitis
        Fatal in 3-6 days

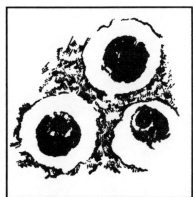

Naegleri fowleri in brain

        Brain -   Swollen/soft
                    Massive vascular congestion
                    Thin exudate
                    Thromboses
        CSF -   Increase in neutrophils
                    Contains blood and amebas
        Affects -   Spinal column, cerebellum
                    Necrosis of grey matter

Course of Disease:
> Burrows through nasal mucosum
> Up olfactory nerve to brain

Diagnosis
> Spinal tap -   cloudy/purulent
>   Increased neutrophils
>   Mobile ameba
>
> Serology -   Indirect florescent antibody test
>
> Hematology -   Increase leucocytes
>   No eosinophilia

Treatment: Called CDC - Atlanta Georgia

Epidemiology:
> Acquire in stagnant warm brackish water
> First described 1965 - over 4 dozen cases - all fatal
> Limited to California, Florida, Georgia, Virginia

NAME OF DISEASE: Amebic meningoencephalitis

Causative Organisms: Acanthemeba
Hartmannella culbersoni
Hartmannella rhysodes

Characteristics of Organism:
Hartmannella -   10-25 micrometers
nuclei sharply defined
dense nucleolus
Acanthameba -   large
spiny multiple pseudopods
double walled cysts

Clinical Symptoms:
Meningoencephalitis -
incubation - 10 days
lesions in brain
focal areas of necrosis
thromboses
affects those with reduced resistance

Eye infection -   Due to homemade contact solutions or
swimming with contacts
Heat will kill cysts
Mild to severe pain
Reduced vision
Enucleation of eye

Complications: Corneal damage

Diagnosis: For eye - scrapings/histology

Treatment: Gentamicin
Sulfadiazine

Epidemiology: First described 1973
Over 100 cases since
Mostly in Arizona, Texas, Louisiana, Florida,
Virginia, Pennsylvania, New York

Ciliophoran Diseases
(Ciliata)

Balantidiasis

largest protozoan

NAME OF DISEASE: Balantidiasis
OTHER NAME(S):   Balantidiosis, Ciliary dysentery,
                     balantidial dysentery, gastroenteritis
                     (general)

Causative Organism: <u>Balantidium</u> <u>coli</u>

Characteristics of Organism:
    Trophozoite stage
        Large, 50-70 micrometers by 40-70 micrometers
        Short numerous cilia embedded in refractile covering
        Water vacuoles clearly visible
        Kidney-bean shaped macronucleus
        Small micronucleus in concavity of macronucleus
        Anaerobic growing
            conditions
        Ingests colonic bacteria

    Cyst stage
        spherical
        Smaller -
            45-65 micro-
                meters
        Double transparent
                wall

<u>Balantidiosis</u> <u>coli</u>
A. Trophoziote
B. Cyst

Portal of Entry:
        fecal-oral route
        contaminated meat, usually pork

Pigs

Clinical Symptoms:
    Nausea/vomiting
    Abdominal colic
    Mild to profuse diarrhea
    Possible ulcers (but not as common as amebiasis
    Mild anemia/mild leucocytosis

Complications:
    Fetal peritonitis

Diagnosis:
    Direct examination of stool. Size makes it easy to see

Treatment:
    Tetracycline   *1st choice*
    Iodoquinol
    Nitrimidazine
    Metronidazole   *2nd*

Epidemiology:
    Reservoir - Pig
    Control Pigs and their manure

MASTIGOPHORAN DISEASES
(FLAGELLATA)

Microsporidiosis
Giardiasis
Trichomoniasis
Trypanosomiasis
Chagas Disease
Cutaneous Leishmaniasis
Mucocutaneous Leishmaniasis
Kala Azar

NAME OF DISEASE: Microsporidiosis

Causative Organism: <u>Microsporidium</u>

Characteristics of Organism:
        obligate intracellular parasite
        spiral flagella

Clinical Symptoms:
        Encephalitis
        Keratitis
        Enteritis

Diagnosis:
    Microscopic -   Period Acid Schiff - positive
                      Polar Flagella

    Serology -   Radioimmunossary (RIA)

NAME OF DISEASE: Giardiasis
OTHER NAME(S):   Giardia enteritis, Beaver fever, lambliasis, gastroenteritis (general)

Causative Organism: <u>Giardia lamblia</u> also called <u>Giardia intestinalis</u>

Characteristics of Organism:

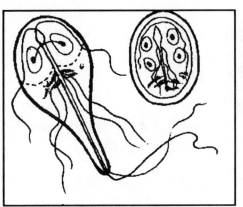

Giardia lamblia -
trophozoile

Trophozoite stage
    Small - 10-18
      micrometers by
      6-11 micro-
        meters
    Four pairs of
      anterior
        flagella
    Two nuclei
    Bilateral
      Symmetry
    Feeds on mucous
    Movement on
      glass slide - as a falling leaf
    Not affect by chlorination
    Small enough to pass through faulty filters
    Adhesive disc used to attached to intestines

    Cyst stage
      About same size
      Wall thickens
      Survives in environment a long time

Portal of Entry: Fecal - oral route

Clinical Symptoms:
    Disease limited to duodenum
    Inflammation, superficial mucosa destruction
    Malabsorption results in greasy, malodorous, pale, loose stools
      (mimics cholecystitis)

Very small
Pair shaped
4 pairs of
flagella

Resistant
alkaline

BEAVERS

grayish

Stools frothy
Flatulence/cramps
Mucous in stool, no blood
Nausea
Itchy rash
Epigastric tenderness

Complications:
Joint inflammation
Reactive arteritis

Diagnosis:
Collecting organism -   Patient swallows gelatin capsule with string 4-8 hours retrieve. Examine for flagellates

Serology - Enterotest for giardia

Treatment:
Quinacrine HCL (Atabrine) and Furazolidone
Metronidazole
Fluid replacement

Epidemiology:
Most common gastroenteritis in United States
Common in Colorado, New York and Pennsylvania
Reservoir - Beavers

odoR in stools.

pain Abdomen

difficult to treat

NAME OF DISEASE: Trichomoniasis

Causative Organism: <u>Trichomonas</u> <u>vaginalis</u>

Characteristics of Organism:
Pear-shapedmastigophoran
No cyst stage
Can survive in warm, moist
    environments
Size - 25 micrometers by
    18 micrometers
Two pair, anterior flagella
    plus one pair laterally
In undulating membrane
Microscopic movement -
    quick, jerky
Thrives in acidic
    environment

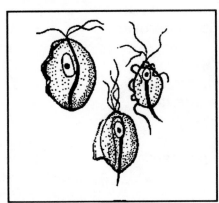
Trichomonads

smaller than Giardia

Predisposition:
Poor hygiene
Diabetes/acidosis
Mechanical contraceptives and spermicides
Decrease in vaginal ph and glucose

chocolat soda increases acid

Portal of Entry:
Genitourinary
Via fomites

Clinical Symptoms:

In male -   Painful urination
    Urethral discomfort
    Possible secondary bacterial invasion
    evident purulent discharge
    (milky discharge)

In female -   Intense itching/burning
    Pururitis
    Internal stinging pain

can cause sterility is already low sperm count

Painful urination

336

Urinary Frequency
Edema
Copious - yellow to clear discharge
 "fishy odor"
Cervicitis/erosion/bleeding

Complications:
    Infertility
    Linked to cervical cancer - dependent on frequency

Diagnosis:
    Microscopic - Examination of urethral discharge
        Gram Stain   Acridine Orange
        Giemsa Stain   Papanicolaou

    Serology -   Immunofluorescence Tests
                 Complement Fixation

Treatment:
    Metronidazole (all partners)
    Tinidazole
    Miconazole
    Floraquin (Diodoquin, boric acid, lactose, dextrose)

estrogen - if post menstrual makes cells so they don't dry out

erodes cervix.

PAP smears

NOTES:

NAME OF DISEASE: Trypanosomiasis
OTHER NAME(S):   African sleeping sickness

Causative Organism: Two varieties
    West African form - <u>Typensoma</u> <u>brucei</u> var <u>gambiense</u>
    East African form - <u>Trypanosoma</u> <u>bruccei</u> var <u>rhodiense</u>

Characteristics of Organism:
    Hemoflagellate about 20
        micrometers
    Four stages of development
        Amastigote - without
           flagella
    Promastigote - single, free,
        anterior   flagella,
        undulating membrane
    Epimastigote - Free anterior
        flagella,   undulating
        membrane
    Trypomastigote - fully mature

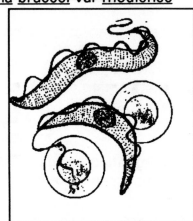

<u>Trypansoma</u> <u>gambiense</u>

Portal of Entry: Bite of <u>Glossina</u> (tsetse fly)
      Unusual characteristics effects
       Spread of disease
             1. Feed by day - netting ineffective
             2. Long - flighted - spread over large
                 areas
             3. Long - lived - up to 3 months
             4. Both male and female are vectors

Clinical Symptoms:

    Three stages to disease
        1. parasitemia
        2. lymphadenitis
        3. Central Nervous System involvement
    Enlarged lymph nodes
    Hepatosplenomegaly
    Posterior cervical triangle lymph nodes enlarged - -
    Winterbottom's sign

Fever/chills
Skin eruptions
Nausea/Vomiting
Slurred/Difficult speech
Disturbed vision
Demyelinating encephalitis
    mental deterioration
    falling asleep
    coma

Rhodesia form - Incubation - weeks, death in months
    Also myocarditis
        edema
        anemia
        secondary bacterial pneumonia

Gambian Form - Incubation - months, death in years

Course of Disease:
    Tsetse fly bites an infected person
    Trypanosomas to insect gut
    Development in gut and salivary glands
    Tsetse fly bites susceptible host
    Development within fly - 2 to 3 weeks

Diagnosis:
    Microscopic -   Aspirates of lymph nodes
                         Blood - Wright's stain
                         CSF in late stages
                         Concentrating of trypanosomas
                             Zinc - sulfate flotation
                             Ritchie - formalin ether method

    Serology - Indirect hemagglutination
                10 fold increase IgM
                ELISA
                Indirect fluorescent antibody test

Treatment:
    Suramin sodium - early stage
    Pentamidine isethionate - hemolymphatic stage
    CNS stage Mel B (Melarsprol)
             Tryparsamide
             Berenilnitrosmidazole

Epidemiology:
    Reservoir   Rhodesian form - human
                Gambian form - animals
                  (problem of control)

    Evades immune system - problem vaccine
            Constantly new parasites with new surface glycoproteins
            15-100 antigens

    Infective dose low - 500 organisms
    250,000 cases 1 year - 20,000 deaths per year

NAME OF DISEASE: Chagas Disease
OTHER NAME(S):   American trypanosomiasis, rangeli

Causative Organism: <u>Trypanosoma</u> <u>cruzi</u>

Characteristics of organism
        Flagellate about 20 micrometers in length
        Single Flagellum
        Similar stages of development as other trypanosomas
            (see Trypanosomiasis)
        Multiply in tissue (not blood)

Portal of entry:
        Break in skin
        Vector - Reduviid bug (triatomid)
            Night feeders
            <u>Triatoma</u> or <u>Rhodinus</u>
            Trypansonosomas in feces
            Self inoculation
            Nickname of bug - kissing bug
            Weak proboscis - bites thin
            skin, like lips
        Ocular rubbing
        Blood transfusion in regions were epidemic

Clinical Symptoms:
        Incubation - 1 to 2 weeks
        Chagoma - hard lesion at site of bite
        3 to 4 centimeters, papular swelling, central red spot
        Disappears in 2 to 3 weeks
        Go lymph nodes, multiply and form aggregates -
            pseudocyst
        Pseudocysts rupture - tissue, necrosis and
            inflammation, organism goes to heart, brain,
            intestines
        Intermittent fever
        Splenomegaly
        Lymphadenopathy
        Joint pain
        Headache

Lethargy
Anorexia
Muscle wasting
Anemia/thrombocytopenia
Dysphagia/Diarrhea

Chronic Affects:

A-V node
tachycardia
hypotension
cardiac enlargement and failure
(pale pink in color)
Meningoencephalitis
apathy/irritability
personality change
tremors
cerebellar ataxia
oscillatory movements of limbs
Affects peristalsis, results in
mesoesophagus
mesocolon

Complications:
Thromboses/embolism
Congenital complications with parasitemia - 1 of 2 die

Diagnosis:
Microscopic -   Stained blood films
                     Tissue biopsy
Cultural -   NNN media (Navy-NacNeal-Nicolls)
Xenodiagnosis -   Use laboratory raised
                     Sterile reduvid bug
                     Let feed on patient
                     2 - 3 weeks later examine bug for
                              trypanosomas
Serology -   Complement - Fixation

Treatment:
    If early -   Nifurtinox
                 Lampit and Rochagan (benzonidazole)
    Later in the disease - no treatment
    Pentamidine isotheonate prophylactic

Epidemiology:
    Epidemic - Central and South American
                Rarely seen in Southeastern U.S.
    2 - 3,000,000 cases in one year
    Reservoir - opossums
               armadillos
               smaller rodents
               possibility dogs and cats
    Experimental vaccine - not available for humans

NAME OF DISEASE: Cutaneous Leishmania
OTHER NAME(S):   Oriental sore, Alleppo button, Delhi boil,
                           Baghdad ulcer, tropical sore

Causative Organism: <u>Leishmania</u> <u>tropia</u>
                           3 varieties - <u>major</u>, <u>minor</u>, <u>aethiopica</u>
                           (diffuse cutaneous leishmaniasis)

Characteristic of Organism:
     Two stage life cycle -
           Amastigote - non
                flagellated
                (In humans)
           Promastigote -
                Flagellated
                (in vector)
     In human -
           live in macrophage
           observed as bipolar -
                staining
           bodies called Donovan
                bodies

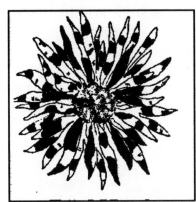

<u>Leishmania</u> <u>tropica</u>
with prominent
Flagella

Portal of Entry:
     Break in skin
     Vector - sand fly (<u>Phlebotomus</u>)

Clinical Symptoms:
     Incubation two to six months
     Inoculated area enlarges/dry scab forms
     Scab falls off
     Severe itching
     heals nine to twelve months
     leaves depigmented scar

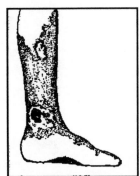

cutaneous
leishmaniasis

Complications:
     Secondary bacterial infections

Diagnosis:

    Microscopic -   Aspirates from ulcer

                        Stain - Giemsa

                                 Leishman

    Serology -   Indirect florescent antibody test

Treatment:

    Neostiban

    Antimony

    Atabarine

    Antibiotics as needed

Epidemiology:

    Reservoir - dogs/dog urine

NAME OF DISEASE: Mucocutaneous Leishmaniasis
OTHER NAME(S):   American Leishmaniasis, uta, espundia

Causative Organism(s): <u>Leishmania</u> <u>braziliansis</u>
                       <u>Leishmania</u> <u>mexicana</u>

Characteristics of Organism:
    See cutaneous Leishmaniasis

Portal of Entry:
    See cutaneous Leishmaniases

Clinical Symptoms:
    Massive tissue necrosis/destruction
    Particularly nasopharyngeest mucosa

Complication:
    Secondary bacterial infection
    Septicemia

Diagnosis:
    See cutaneous Leishmaniasis

Treatment:
    Lampit
    Neostiban
    Antimony

NAME OF DISEASE: Kala Azar
OTHER NAME(S):   Black- Fever, Dum-Dum Fever
                  Splenic anemia (infants)

Causative Organism: Leishmania donovani

Characteristics of Organism:
    See cutaneous Leishmaniasis

Portal of entry:
    Break in skin
    Vector - sand fly (Phlebotomus)
    Also - nasal secretions
           urine
           feces

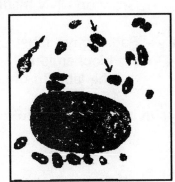

Donovan bodies - large structure nucleus of phagocyte

Clinical Symptoms:
    Infection of reticulo - endothelial
        system
    Destroys macrophage and other
        phagocytes
    Depresses host defense mechanism
    Fever
    Skin turns dark
    Lymphadenopathy
    Progressive anemia
    Edema - which may mask emaciation
    Leukopenia
    Bleeding gums
    Hepatosplenomegaly

Complications:
    Uncontrollable hemorrhage
    Dysentery
    Septicemia
    Pneumonia/TB
    Dermal leishmaniasis - resembles lepromatous
        Hansen's disease

Diagnosis:

    Microscopic -   Liver/spleen aspirates
                                   Stain - Leishman
                                      Giemsa

    Cultural -   Grow on NNN media or Chang media

    Rediorespirametry - Radioactive label coupled with unique biochemistry. Observe uptake of the label in the organism

    Skin test -   Sensitivity - Montenegro's

Treatment: Pentamidine

SPOROZOAL DISEASES

Malaria
Toxoplasmosis
Pneumocytosis

NAME OF DISEASE: Malaria

Causative Organism: Various species of <u>Plasmodium</u>

Characteristics of Organism:
    Multiple stage life cycle
    Schizogony (in human host)
        Sporozoites introduce by bite of mosquito
        Within ½ hour disappear from blood in liver
        Exoerythrocytic stage -
            various stages of schizont
            until merozoites formed
        Erythrocytic stage -
            merozoites invade RBC
            form trophozoite
            mitosis/cytoplasmic segmentation
            schizont reform
            change to merozoites
            release and infect other RBC's
    Sporogony (in mosquito)
        Sometimes merozoites change into macrogametocyte and microgametocyte. They become microgamete and macrogamete which become sperm and egg. Fertilization creates ookinete. Ookinete attaches to insects gut, forms oocyst. Ruptures, releasing sporozoites
    Cycle repeats

Portal of entry: Break in skin
                  Vector - <u>Anopheles</u> Mosquito

Clinical Symptoms:
    Paroxysmal set of symptoms - cycle 48-72 hours
    Shaking/chills (15-20 minute)
    Headache
    Vomiting
    Lasts 1-2 hours
    Rapid rise in temperature - 104°-106°F
    Lasts 3 to 4 hours

Massive perspiration
Lasts 2 to 4 hours
Or a total of 6 to 10 hours and repeated at regular intervals
Other symptoms:
        hypochromic, microcytic anemia
        hypertrophy of liver, darkened
        enlarged, fibrotic spleen, darkened
        RES hyperplasia
        Leukopenia - 20% reduction in monocytes
        Increase of hemoglobin breakdown products
        Flaciparum Form - blood sticky
                        capillary occlusion
                        in brain - cerebral malaria
"Blackwater Fever" -   hemoglobinuric nephrosis
                        black urine

Course of Disease:
        Anopheles bites host, feeds, salivates
        Saliva introduces sporozoites
        Infective dose over 500,000
        Go to liver
        6 - 9 days later released
        Merozoites in blood - next uncontaminated   mosquito that
            feeds continues cycle

Complications:
        encephala
        hemiplegia
        convulsions
        coma
        congestive heart failure
        pulmonary edema
        renal failure

Diagnosis:
        Microscopic -   Blood smears
                      Identify signet ring form in RBC
                      Used absolute alcohol fixture
                      2-3 minutes followed by giemsa

Screening -   SAFA - soluble antigen fluorescent
                           antibody test
History of travel

Hematology -   decreased hemoglobin
                   decreased WBC

Treatment:
Prophylactic: Quinine sulfate
              Fansidor (sulfadiazine/pyrimethamine)
Acute: Chloroquine (aroilen)
Liver: Primaquine
Others: Chlorguanide
              Mefloquine - (resistant strains)

Epidemiology:
    4 species of Plasmodium
        P. falciparum - most serious
                         causes malignant subtertcian
                             malaria (estivo-autumnal)
                         cycle varies 36-72 hours
        P. vivax -   causes benign tertian malaria
                         cycle - 48 hours
        P. malariae -   quartan malaria
                         cycle - 72 hours
        P. ovale -   tertian malaria
                         cycle - 48 hours

Control - insecticides - DDT, lindane, dieldrin
          destroy larvae
          oil in water where larvae develop - prevents breathing
          drain swamps
          biological - introduce fish that eat larvae or mosquitoes

NAME OF DISEASE: Toxoplasmosis

Causative Organism: <u>Toxoplasma gondii</u>

Characteristics of Organism:
    Obligate intracellular parasite
    Sexual stage in mammal, mainly
      cat
    Forms oocysts - released in feces
      (oocyst contains eight
        infectious sporozoites)
    Viable for about 1 year in
      environment
    In humans - two stages
      tachyzoites - feeding form
      bradyzoites - conglomeration
    Crescent shape - 4-7 micrometers by 2-4 micrometers
    Tachyzoite easily killed by physical agents

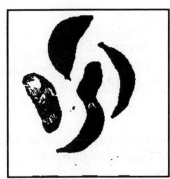

<u>Toxoplasma gondii</u>

Portal of Entry:
    Oral
    Congenital

Clinical Symptoms:
    Congenital - hydrocephalus/microcephalus
            cerebral calcification
            encephalomyelitis
            liver enlargement
            skin rash/yellow coloration
            retardation
            blindness
            epilepsy

    Localized Toxoplasmosis -   fever
                       lymphadenopathy
                       mononucleosis-like
                          symptoms

Generalized Toxoplasmosis - encephalitis (children)
                            fever
                            delirium/convulsions
                            maculopapular rash

Complications: hepatitis
                myocarditis
                pneumonitis
                polymyositis

Diagnosis:
    Microscopic - sputum, vaginal aspirates
                  air-dry/giemsa

    In Vivo -   inject mice with patient tissue
                 (I.P.)
                 incubate 5-10 days
                 organisms in mice peritoneal fluid

    Serology -   complement fixation
                 Sabin-Feldman dye test--
                     patient serum + T. gondii
                     stain methylene blue
                     serum prevents staining - positive
                 ELISA Test

Treatment: Triple sulfa and pyrimethamine (sulfadiazine,
    sulfamerazine, sulfamethazine and pyrimethamine)

Epidemiology:
    Sources of infection - raw meat (pick up cysts while
                           grazing)
                           cats - via prey that is infected
                           fomites - litter box

    1 in a 1,000 babies born with congenital toxoplasmosis or
        3,000-4,000 children a year.

NAME OF DISEASE: Pneumocytosis pneumonia

Causative Organism: <u>Pneumocytosis</u> <u>carinii</u>

Characteristics of Organism:
    Cysts -   4-10 microcrometes, round
                1-8 sporozoites
    Trophozoite - 2-5 micrometers
                V-shaped nuclear material
                Crescent - shaped
                Killed by macrophages unless faulty immune
                    system
                Multiply in alveoli

Portal of Entry: Inhalation
                    Direct Contact

Clinical Symptoms:
    4-6 week course of infection
    cough - productive/non-productive
    shortness of breath/tachypnea
    cyanosis
    intermittent fever
    atelectasis - consolidation viewed on x-ray
    alveoli - foamy exudate, lightly stained, organisms present
              and inflammatory cells

Complications: pneumothorax
                  pneumodiastinum
                  pulmonary fibrosis

Diagnosis:
    Microscopic - biopsy material
              stain - Gomori methemine silver
                    Toluidine blue
                    Papanicolaou
                    Gram - Wiegart
                    Gridley

Treatment: Trimethoprim
                Sulfamethoxazole
                Pyrimethamine
                Trisulfapyridine
                Pentamidine
                Plus -   oxygen
                              supportive due to hypoxia

OTHER PROTOZOAL DISEASES

Babesiosis
Crytosporidiosis
Isosporiasis
Sarcocytosis
Heliobacter Gastritis

NAME OF DISEASE: Babesiosis
OTHER NAME(S):   Piroplasmosis, Red Water Fever (cattle)

Causative Organism - <u>Babesia</u> <u>microtia</u>

Characteristics of Organism:
    appear ameboid
    round to rod shaped
    1-5 micrometers

Portal of Entry: Break in skin
                     Vector-tick (<u>Ixodes</u>)

Clinical Symptoms:
    High fever/chills
    piercing headache
    muscle pain
    mild anemia
    dark urine
    hemoglobinuria/hemoglobinemia
    Jaundice
    Renal failure
    Capillary occlusions

Treatment: Chloroquine

Epidemiology -   Can be confused with Falciparum malaria, but
                         differences
                     No blood breakdown pigments
                     No exoerythrocytic stage
                     No sexual stage
                     Mostly in coastal Massachusetts and
                         Long Island
                     Most severe in those with splenectomy
                     Problem for blood banking - can be
                         transmitted via blood

NAME OF DISEASE: Cryptosporidiosis

Causative Organisms: <u>Cryptosporidium</u>

Portal of Entry: Fecal-Oral route

Clinical Symptoms:
    Asymptomatic
    Incubation - 4-12 days
    Mild infection -   24 hour stomach flu
                  headache
                  sweating
                  vomiting
                  cramps/diarrhea
    Immune-compromised (AIDS) -
            severe diarrhea
            up to 25 bowel movements/day
            up to 17 liters/days
            malabsorption
            infection of ileum-cecum
            prominent peyer's patches
            draining lymph nodes
            eroded villi

Epidemiology:
    First described 1976 - water contaminated by cattle feces
    Opportunistic infection
    Possible source - puppies/kittens

NAME OF DISEASE: Isosporiasis
OTHER NAME(S):   Coccidiosis

Causative Organism: <u>Isosporium</u> <u>belli</u>

Characteristics of Organism:
      oocysts - double walled
              ellipsoid

Portal of Entry: Oral

Clinical Symptoms:
      Acute or chronic diarrhea
      Characterized - fever
                  diarrhea/cramps
                  peripheral eosinophilia
      Effects small intestine - mucosal atrophy - malabsorption

Diagnosis:
      Microscopic: biopsy
                 oocyst in stools

Treatment: Sulfonamide

NAME OF DISEASE: Sarcocytosis

Causative Organism: <u>Sarcocytosis bovihominis</u>
                      <u>Sarcocytosis suishominis</u>

Characteristics of Organism:
    Gametes fuse in animal host
    Forms cyst
    Released in human
    forms 2 sporocysts with 4 sporozoites
    Go to endothelium form merozoites
    To muscle to become bradyzoites
    Forming intranuclear cysts

Clinical Symptoms:
    nausea
    abdominal pain
    diarrhea

Epidemiology:
    Reservoir - pigs/cows

NAME OF DISEASE: Heliobacter gastritis

Causative Organism: <u>Heliobacter</u> <u>pylori</u>

Portal of Entry: Oral

Clinical Symptoms:

  Duodenal ulcers
  Inflammation of intestinal mucosa

Treatment:
  Bismuth
  Metronidazole

Algal Disease

Paralytic Shellfish Poisoning

NAME OF DISEASE: Paralytic Shellfish Poisoning
OTHER NAME(S):   PSP

Causative Organism: <u>Gonyaulax</u> <u>cataenella</u>

Characteristics of Organism:
    Class <u>Pyrrophcophyta</u> (<u>Pyrrophyta</u>)
        A dinoflagellate
        Warm, marine algae
        Pigments - phycoerythrin
        Colors ocean when overgrows - (blooms) called red
            tide
        Blooms warmer months
        Concentration of over 200 cells/ml of surrounding
        water - algae produces enough toxin to contaminate
        fish and their flesh and thereby people

Portal of entry:
    Oral
    Mostly shellfish which concentrate via manner of ingestion

Clinical Symptoms:
    Toxin affects CNS
    Temporary paralysis of extremities

Diagnosis:
    Clinical end patient history

Treatment:
    Symptomatic